THOUSANDS OF PEOPLE CHANGES TO THEIR CO BY APPLYING THE POW~~ERFUL STRATEGIES AND~~ MATERIAL IN THIS BOOK!

Andrew has done such a great job laying out his content and insights in a pithy but engaging fashion. There's no fluff but there is a great manner in the voice in which he writes. No self-congratulatory preachy-ness, no hype, just the sense of an honorable mission to convince me that he has trod a path, maybe similar to mine, and he can tell me what tools and methods he used. I have had some experience with neurolinguistic practitioners, therapists, and executive coaches--and books--and recognize the breadth of learning, personal experience and interaction with the material that filtered into this book. It meshes nicely with the content and insights I've been given in coaching programs from experts costing thousands of dollars. Definitely a re-read. The book delivers as advertised.

DAVE CASTRO / USA

This book is incredible when it comes to finding the issues that we have been taught and or learned from observation that has formed our concepts of getting the most out of life and becoming the most that is possible in our lives. Andrew starts out with the very basics of a child's learning and discovery process that we all go through. So much of what we have been taught growing up is false in terms of leading the life that was designed in us from the very beginning. He teaches how to recognize these false concepts and beliefs and then how to make the correct changes that ultimately has the potential to change our flawed way of thinking of ourselves to a way that will enable a person to see themselves in a more rewarding and growing way of thinking.

GENE ERWIN / USA

This is not just any ordinary self-development book. If you are truly seeking to improve your self-confidence than I highly recommend this read. Andrew has included step by step instructions on how to change your mindset. Learning how to quiet your ego is no easy task but after reading this book I have absolutely more power and skills to live a more product life on my terms. I am excited to incorporate my new found abilities and self-confidence into all aspects of my life.

HEENA DANNA / USA

Andrew Leedham presents some thought-provoking ideas in this refreshing, no-frills, honest approach to resetting and reprogramming one's thoughts and perceptions. As humans, we are by-products of the society we interact in and as a result, a lot of people become what their peers think of them. Andrews's approach, coupled with an internal "makeover" and ridding oneself of the bad programming leads to a better self-image and in turn, *Unstoppable Self Confidence*. 5/5, the best book I have read on the subject.

MARC KOBRIN / USA

I've been a student of personal development for many years and have found many 'tools' to help progress in this journey of life, but I am so grateful to Andrew Leedham for THIS book! It is different from everything else out there! He not only helps us truly identify the real stuff that has been holding us back in such a simple, yet powerful way but he helps us create new programming that is fast and permanent (my friend who recommended the book to me is proof of this!). Andrew came from rock-bottom and was a 'regular' guy (not a guru in self-help stuff) who applied these strategies in his own life and experienced the incredible transformation that IS the foundation of his life now. And the cool thing is that we ALL have everything we need to do the same. I'm feeling the transition in myself (so excited) and wish I had this book years ago! It's so good and easy to connect with, I gave my 21-year-old son a copy and he's already started taking the journey. I can only imagine what he will do in this world with the right programming found in *Unstoppable Self Confidence!* Thank you, Andrew!

KRISTI KOZEL / CANADA

I love this book, its well thought out, clearly and succinctly written. I can feel it actually changing me as I do the work, the work is not difficult, it's interesting and does not feel punishing, instead it feels releasing and beneficial. Andrew is a genius. I am also doing a live course with him and his live training is also fantastic. A great buy.

HELEN F / UK

An incredible accumulation of wisdom that I had never seen before in one book, dealing with how WE have the power to take back control of our minds and stop allowing other peoples' opinions, events around us, and most importantly, our own "self-programming" to continue to hold us back from living our awesome lives to the fullest. Our only limits are those limits we allow to exist. Andrew has done a fabulous job of providing you great tools to release those limiting beliefs and take back control of your thoughts! Not new material, but a great accumulation of masters...it will change your life for the better!! And don't expect to absorb it in one reading...maybe 5! But start putting it in practice immediately!

LYDIA STASIAK / USA

This is quite simply the best self-help book I have ever read, and I have read a lot! From the first few words that we are not broken it is comforting, realistic, and practical. Easy to follow Andrew guides and prompts action. It has transformed my internal world which has impacted massively on my outer world. I would urge anyone who is looking to make changes in their life to not waste a moment elsewhere, this book is where you need to be. It is like coming home.

ALISON BARCLAY / UK

Read this book. Read it again. More importantly apply the fundamental lessons in this book regularly and you will see a dramatic shift in your outlook and mindset in a very short space of time. Whatever time you put in your rewards will be tenfold. As an avid reader of mindset books this is by far the one that has had the most impact.

S C WILCOX / UK

UNSTOPPABLE
SELF
CONFIDENCE

HOW TO CREATE THE INDESTRUCTIBLE,
NATURAL CONFIDENCE OF THE 1% WHO
ACHIEVE THEIR GOALS, CREATE SUCCESS
ON DEMAND AND LIVE LIFE
ON THEIR TERMS

ANDREW LEEDHAM

WHAT THIS BOOK CAN DO
for you

This book is all about how to create the indestructible, natural confidence and success of the 1% - the 1% of people who live life on their terms and achieve success in all they do.

In this no-nonsense, application-specific guide, I'll be giving you the most powerful strategies and success principles to build the mindset and confidence that will make you ***completely unstoppable.***

Most importantly, the way I teach this to you is what makes the transformation of your confidence ***permanent***.

The problem is that most teaching on confidence and success is completely back to front, and so it either doesn't work or causes way, way, way more problems than it solves.

The way most books teach confidence and success means that even though most of those books contain genuinely great material, it isn't presented in a way that allows you to access the incredible value they hold.

These differences are crucial in your journey to becoming who you want to be and to creating the life you want to live.

Here's just some of what you'll learn in this book:

- **How to switch back on the natural confidence you had as a child**
- How to silence the negative voice in your head
- **Discover the secret techniques to control your confidence on demand**
- How to stop caring what other people think
- **Learn the system to break free from your limiting beliefs**
- How to get in control of your mind
- **The two core questions that define everyone's confidence**
- Revealed: How to eliminate worry, fear and anxiety forever
- **The secret traps that keep you feeling bad about yourself**
- The secret method for actually getting what you desire in life

This book is dedicated to my two incredible daughters, Lara and Ava. They inspire me every day and simply light up my world.

Two other people I must thank are Andy Shaw and Stephen Hedger.

Andy and his Saltori Structured Thinking System gave me the blueprint for a life that works. He opened my eyes to a completely different way of thinking and living and showed me the path.

Stephen is the most gifted relationship coach in the world today. During my darkest time he showed me who I could be, the man I could become.

This book contains numerous insights and inspirations from them both.

And to my family, who never gave up on me.

To Lara, Ava, Andy and Stephen, Mum and Dad, Katherine and Greg, I am more grateful than you know.

CONTENTS

STEP ONE

HOW TO PRIME YOUR MINDSET FOR INCREDIBLE SUCCESS

STEP TWO

HOW TO REMOVE THE BAD PROGRAMMING THAT'S HOLDING YOU BACK

IMPORTANT NOTE

HOW TO USE THIS BOOK TO TRANSFORM YOUR CONFIDENCE, PERMANENTLY

This book is divided into four parts. Although you may be tempted to flick through it and go straight to the sections that apply to you most, you should, when you've finished flicking, read the whole book in order.

Why? Because this book has been designed to **take you on the journey you need** to transform how you see yourself and how you feel about who you are, permanently.

Lots of books can show you plenty of techniques and tricks to make you **feel good**. But this book is about **change that lasts**.

My goal for you, is that by reading this book, we alter the direction of your life, that you come to see the greatness within you, and we set you on the path of living the life you've always dreamed of.

I understand that might seem impossible now, but just for now, don't judge. Instead decide to trust the process.

Each section of the book is a building block, that gives you what you need **in the right order** to unleash your natural confidence.

By jumping ahead, you risk feeling better for a while and then falling back into your old patterns of thinking. Then despite the fact that you have found the answer you're looking for, it will seem like you haven't.

Sometimes it's better to follow the instruction manual!

This book gives you:

Step 1 provides the core foundations to unlock your natural confidence and a revealing understanding of how you went on the journey to losing the natural confidence and successful thinking you were born with. **Step 2** shows you the bad teaching that has bent your thinking out of shape and shut down your natural confidence and success mindset. I'll show you the proven, time-tested strategies and techniques to remove – for good – the crooked thinking patterns that are holding you back. **Step 3** gives you the powerful transformative techniques, strategies, and ways of thinking of the top 1%. You will see what they do to live with unstoppable self-confidence and to create incredible success, no matter the goal, situation, or challenge – and why this makes them virtually certain to succeed. You'll learn not only what these techniques are, but also how to install them permanently in your mindset. Now you've transformed your thinking, **Step 4** shows you how to generate results in your life fast and how to deal with any challenges that arise along the way.

Commit to applying the strategies in this book. They work!

Here's what I suggest: underline every passage that is important to you as you read it. Scientific tests have shown that when you underline a passage, you absorb information two or three times more effectively.

Second, take a break at the end of each chapter and consider the questions and notes raised in the final section of each chapter. Despite what you may think, this is where you will get the most benefit. As you go through each question or point, think of an example from your own life where the question or point applies. By understanding clearly how you're not applying the right thinking today, you will get the biggest results most quickly.

Lastly, and most importantly, you'll be surprised at how little I actually talk about confidence in this book. *This is entirely on purpose.* The problem with focusing on confidence is that it requires energy to sustain it. Over time this will exhaust you and you will inevitably fall back into your old thinking patterns.

Instead, I'm teaching you how to be **naturally confident and successful**, which happens when **no direct effort is applied** to trying to be confident.

By learning the thought structures, the **mindset**, of the 1%, confidence happens as a byproduct and requires no energy at all to sustain it. **And that's why it lasts**. For things to last, they have to come naturally.

FREE GIFT

As a thank you for buying this book I'd like to offer you <u>free access</u> to some courses and ebooks that are **so good they transform your confidence on demand.** You can get them here: www.unstoppableselfconfidence.com/confidence-on-demand

---

THE JOURNEY BACK

The words hit me like a hammer: "There's nothing wrong with you. You're not broken; you never were. So you don't need fixing. You've simply lost your way. And I'm here to show you the way back. And it's not difficult or complicated."

I was sitting in the office of my coach, Stephen, at probably the lowest point in my life. My marriage was over; I was facing a toxic, difficult divorce.

I was desperately worried about my two beautiful little girls whose world was being turned upside down. And I was facing losing my family, my relationship, my home, and potentially nearly all my time with my children.

And that was on top of knowing that there was a high chance that financially I would lose everything I had worked incredibly hard to build up over the previous 15 years.

But far more importantly, I knew I had completely lost myself. I no longer knew who I was outside of my marriage, outside of being a father, outside of the world that was now being torn apart.

My whole sense of who I was and what gave me purpose was disintegrating.

When you suddenly lose so much that defines who you are and what your life is, it can be an incredibly daunting, dark, scary place to be. Yet that is exactly where I found myself.

Everything that felt at one time so certain and clear becomes unstable and shaky.

For so much of my life I'd had bulletproof confidence.

I knew who I was and liked who I was. I'd achieved some incredible things, been financially very successful, had great relationships, great friends and family, and had had amazing adventures. I'd achieved my dream of becoming a millionaire. I knew what I wanted and where I was going in life. I felt good, *really good*, about myself.

I liked being me.

Yet now, I felt like a shell of that person, hollowed out and empty. As my marriage had deteriorated, I'd progressively given up more and more of myself and what mattered to me to try to save our relationship and keep our family together.

I didn't like – in fact, I felt deeply ashamed – of who I had become. I felt that there was something fundamentally and *uniquely* wrong with me. That if people saw who I really was underneath the shell they would be horrified.

I started to notice little things that really bothered me, and deep down I knew something was badly wrong. I noticed that I didn't like to look in the mirror or see photos of myself. I felt disconnected from the person looking back at me; that person always looked somehow wrong, different from everyone else and somehow out of place.

I didn't respect myself. How could I? I was living against almost every value that mattered to me, that defined who I was. To hold my marriage together, I was making decisions that I knew were wrong and that I really didn't like.

I'd stopped taking care of myself and given up on my passions and interests. All the things that made me who I was.

My time, my thoughts, my life were almost entirely about doing things for others.

I no longer bothered arguing with people when they behaved badly towards me. In truth I didn't feel there was any point. I didn't feel that I deserved any better.

Most of the therapists that we had seen during the last stages of our marriage had only succeeded in making it worse. They had, in the process, made me feel awful, and deeply inadequate as a husband, as a man, and as an individual.

I remember thinking that if everything that those therapists had told me was true, then there was so much wrong with me that there wasn't enough time left in my life to fix it all.

That all that was left for me was a huge amount of effort to make my life, make me, <u>slightly less broken</u> than I was.

I sat in the chair looking at Stephen, wondering how the hell I had come to this point. How had I ended up in this situation, emptied out, with no passion, no energy, no nothing?

I looked back at photos of me in the past, from before my marriage, seeing the energy, passion, and confidence in my eyes; seeing the possibilities and potential in that person; seeing their excitement about life.

I remembered how easy life felt, how straightforward it seemed; how life seemed full of open doors, exciting people to meet, and incredible adventures to have.

Where had that person gone? Could they ever come back or was it too late for me? Had my time come and gone already before I had even realized?

Stephen calmly listened to all these thoughts tumble out, an unfiltered stream of consciousness.

He then just looked at me and smiled, wisely, calmly, and kindly and said those words that changed everything for me: "There's nothing wrong with you and there never was. Let me show you why."

That was the turning point.

Over the next three months I went on an incredible journey where I completely rebuilt myself. My confidence went from an all-time low to being completely indestructible.

Alongside working with Stephen, my great friend and mentor Andy Shaw was emailing me regularly. He coached me through my divorce, helped me regain control of my mind, and worked with me to get out of my own way. He showed me the mindset of the 1%.

By working with Stephen and Andy together, my journey back to confidence turned from decades into days.

My passion and my energy were completely rejuvenated. I fell back in love with who I was. This wasn't arrogance, just a calm, kind, and deep love for myself. I loved being me again. I felt a calmness and a peace that I hadn't had for years. I knew with a profound certainty that no matter what happened, I was OK and would be just fine.

It took another 12 months to work through my divorce.

Despite all the challenges, the obvious anger, losing my marriage, and the end of my family as a unit – despite losing nearly everything I had spent the previous 15 years building up – and despite the legal challenges and legal bills of a very toxic divorce battle, I was able to just calmly and peacefully observe it all, knowing I would be fine. In fact, better than fine. I actually felt far better than I had in years.

How?

I had regained and reconnected with my natural confidence and success mindset. The one we are all born with, *including you.*

I had dropped all the bullshit negative illusions and self-limiting beliefs that had kept me trapped in a vicious cycle of negative thinking, bad feelings, and low confidence.

All the self-judgement, all the dispiriting self-talk that kept me playing small and trapped. The sense that there was something horribly and uniquely flawed about me, that I was somehow different from everyone else, just fell away.

I had reprogrammed my mind into a powerful, perfectly functioning machine for confidence, growth, and success. I realized I had used this incredible machine between my ears to create all the bad stuff in my life. Now I was going to use it to create all the good stuff again.

The whole experience became a journey of incredible learning. It allowed me to learn, from Stephen and Andy, how I had gone on the journey from incredible confidence and success to being at rock bottom and back again.

This time I wanted to make sure I knew where things could go wrong, what pitfalls I had fallen into, and where I had taken the wrong turns. Never again did I want to, by accident or design, fall into the negative, destructive thinking that had led me to feel so awful, so worthless, so uniquely wrong.

Through this process, through these two brilliant, wonderful mentors, I discovered the blueprint for creating indestructible, unstoppable self-confidence and incredible success. And most importantly, I learned how to stay there permanently.

And that's the blueprint I'm going to show you.

Enjoy this journey. It's wonderful.

INTRODUCTION

> **Maybe the reason nothing seems to be "fixing you" is because you're not broken.**
>
> DR. STEVE MARABOLI

You were born naturally confident.

And despite what you may currently think, being confident is your natural, default state.

Contrary to what most people will tell you, being confident, feeling great about who you are and being able to effortlessly achieve everything you want in life isn't difficult. It is simply a matter of doing the right things in the right order.

It is a process.

The problem is that so much teaching on confidence is backwards.

Fundamentally, you only need to grasp one simple - *but critical* - principle in order to create the natural, indestructible confidence of the 1% who achieve their goals, create success in whatever they do, and live life on their terms.

Nothing can stop your progress once you integrate this foundational principle into your thinking.

It is this:

> **There's nothing wrong with you and *you don't need fixing*. You already have everything you need to be confident and to live exactly the life you want. You only need to UNLEARN all the bad programming and incorrect thinking you've been given to unleash the incredible power within you.**

Take a moment and think about this. A newborn baby has no sense that it doesn't deserve love, care, or attention. A young child learning to walk or learning a language for the first time has no sense that it can't be done. No baby when it sees new people for the first time, has any notion that it is somehow, in some way, not good enough or less than other babies. They don't have any sense that they somehow don't deserve what they want.

That's because those thoughts aren't natural. ***They are learned.***

When you grasp this truth, you realize that any sense of lack you have about who you are and what you can achieve <u>is unnatural and the result of bad teaching</u>.

You realize that any lack of confidence isn't because of who you are. <u>It is because of what you have been taught.</u>

The unconscious and incorrect assumption that we nearly all have is that that our education from our parents, teachers and peers is there to help us – that what we are taught what we need to succeed in life.

But what if that isn't true?

If it was true, then surely more than 1% of people would live the lives they really wanted rather than the lives they have settled for - lives of frustration and quiet desperation.

So perhaps the most surprising - and exhilarating – suggestion I want to put to you is this:

You always have been, and you always will be, in total control of your confidence and results in life.

When I say this to people, they nearly always protest and reel off all the "reasons" why they feel the way they do and can't get the life they want: they don't have much money; they're not as good-looking as someone else; they don't have the job or the connections that someone else has; they don't have time, and hundreds more just like it.

Of course, they're correct, right?

Wrong.

I will show you, no matter what your life looks like today and no matter your personal circumstances, how you can transform your self-esteem and your results in life, FAST.

When you learn to re-connect with your core, when you learn to let go of bullshit thinking and bad programming, when you apply the same natural success thinking that the 1% never lost, your success in life becomes **predictable and inevitable**.

My goal in writing this book is to give you all the precise tools, techniques, and strategies - the exact step by step process - that will give you the indestructible, unstoppable self-confidence and mindset that will transform your results in life from run-of-the-mill to runaway success; from a life of missed opportunities and unfulfilled potential to incredible and certain success; from being at the mercy of events to striding out and putting a huge dent in the universe.

Your dent in the universe.

If that sounds good, then you're really going to enjoy what this book is going to show you.

But there are a couple of other things – **and they are important**.

First, many, in fact most, of the concepts, methods and strategies you'll learn in this book, go against "traditional" teaching and wisdom.

You won't learn these techniques in the vast majority of self-help books or from most therapists.

So I ask you to keep your mind open. As you read through the pages of this book, decide for now **not to judge**, but instead to simply consider what is said.

Your current thinking has brought you to where you are today. Different thinking will take you to the life you want. That thinking is contained in these pages, but it will grate against some or a lot of what you currently "know" to be true.

Your ego (that negative voice in your head) will look to instantly dismiss the new concepts. It will say to you that you "already know this," or that "everybody knows [insert common thought here] is true." When these moments happen, slow down and consider things carefully. You can always judge and dismiss later, but for a few minutes just allow yourself to explore what is being said.

Your ego is also likely to tell you pretty frequently that while some people could achieve the results I talk about, you can't.

This is a lie, a trick that your mind plays on you to keep you stuck. Don't make the mistake of believing it. When this happens, allow yourself to realize the truth that you are not so special **that this work will for everyone else except you**.

You deserve the chance to live the life that you want. Allow yourself to dwell on the real possibilities for your life. You have most likely spent many years focused on what you believe to be the impossibilities. So, just for a little while, give yourself a break from that way of thinking. You can always go back to it later.

Second, you will notice as you read through the book that I repeat myself. I do this **on purpose.**

My sole aim for you is that by reading this book you unleash the natural confidence and success within you, and you get the life you really want.

Most books tell you things once and then wrongly assume that because you've read it, you know it. This is one of the reasons that so many self-help books fail to bring about any lasting change.

There's a famous quote by Will Durant that says, "**We are what we repeatedly do. Excellence then is not an act but a habit.**"

What this means for you is that simply reading this material won't get you the results you want.

What *will get you the results* you want is reading it, then considering the points raised, then (and most importantly) **applying the techniques and strategies**. Rinse and repeat.

That is the model for human learning and mastery of any skill. It doesn't work unless you do all the elements. Just doing some won't help you, just as building some parts of a house doesn't really help you.

So, as you notice the repetition in the book, use it as a prompt, a nudge, to look and see whether you have really understood, and most importantly, whether you have applied and mastered a concept, or if you only think you have mastered it.

There's a very big difference.

All the limits to our lives come from the false assumptions we have allowed in our minds. As you continue to look at these false assumptions again and again, they simply dissolve and you see them for the illusions that they are.

At that point, you remove the hidden blocks that hinder you from achieving your dreams.

So, are you ready for something different?

Let's now get straight on with unleashing your unstoppable natural confidence.

HOW TO PRIME YOUR MINDSET FOR INCREDIBLE SUCCESS

CHAPTER 1

THE KEY TO UNLOCKING YOUR NATURAL SUCCESS MINDSET

Dare to be wrong about who you think you are.

LIZ IVORY

What if I told you that there's nothing wrong with you? That you're not broken and you don't need fixing?

That actually the opposite is true and that you are naturally confident and successful? And all that's happened is that you have been taught, programmed, and socially conditioned by a series of damaging and limiting thoughts that block your <u>natural success mindset and confidence</u> dead in its tracks?

The reason that nothing has seemed to "fix you" is because you've been coming at the real problem backwards.

Because you don't need to load more information, more programming, more conditioning into your mind.

You need to do exactly the opposite.

You, instead, need to **unlearn** all of the limiting, toxic thinking that stops your natural confidence and success mindset from operating in the way it is designed to.

Most mainstream personal development says that you need to change who you are in order to feel good and become confident and successful.

This is not only wrong, but deeply damaging. Let's look at that a little more closely to understand why.

The underlying premise of that teaching is that you need to become something different from who you are in order to be better, successful, liked, and loved.

What that tells a person who is already feeling shitty about themselves is that their fear that they were not good enough just became a fact.

So now you feel worse than you did before, even further away from your dreams than you already thought you were. And you feel somehow defective in a way that confident, successful people are not.

So you read more books, enroll in more courses, and push yourself harder and harder in order to fix yourself and get better.

But each book or course tells you more things "that you are not." More things that you have to become. So again, you feel even further from where you want to be.

Each book reveals more things you have wrong, more things you have to work on, and more ways that you have fallen short of who you need to be to feel confident and live the life you want.

So your efforts to help yourself are now not only **not helping** you but are **actively working against you**. And so each book reveals what appears to be an answer but in fact is only information that ends up sending you backwards. You feel worse and worse, not better and more confident.

Yes, you need to be different from the person you've become, but you don't need to change **_away from_** who you are. You need to change **_back to_** who you **_really_** are.

THE JOURNEY BACK TO NATURAL CONFIDENCE

Let me explain.

Hard-coded deep into your DNA at the point you were conceived, and running through every cell in your body, is an incredible, battle-hardened program to achieve virtually any goal that you can conceive.

This program was loaded onto the most powerful, astonishing supercomputer known to exist anywhere: the human brain. This machine is capable of processing nearly incalculable amounts of information, while simultaneously handling a vast number of complex tasks with incomplete and often incorrect information. And yet, despite this, it can still come up with exactly the right answer.

The human mind – **your mind** – is a miracle.

Your basic, foundational core programming is incredible. Think of a newborn baby: Do they have any sense that they are not worthy? That they shouldn't get what they want? That they can't do something, be something, have something?

You have to learn these limits; it is not your natural way of thinking.

The people who are "naturally" confident and successful are no different from anyone else. They simply, by accident or design, didn't take on this backwards, muddled thinking that holds back 99% of people.

Realizing this and, more importantly, living it, changes everything. Instead of thinking you have to become something you're not, you understand that all you need to do is reconnect with who you really are.

It's a very different journey and one that feels right and natural instead of difficult and hard.

And that small change makes all the difference in the world.

The 1% simply failed to fail. They realized that the rules they were being given didn't work and didn't make sense.

THE WRONG BLUEPRINT

On top of the bad programming of not being good enough, worthy enough, talented enough, or good-looking enough comes layer up on layer of expectation and constraint about who you "should" be, what you "should" want, and what life you "should" live.

So now you've had your natural talents and confidence blunted and then you're set off in the direction of a life of "success" that isn't your own – one where even if you succeed in getting "there," you've failed because it isn't the life you consciously chose. It is the life others chose for you.

So consider, do you live life on your own terms, or someone else's?

Consider that for a moment. Don't just answer straightaway. There's huge value for you in understanding this.

Ask yourself honestly: Is the life you are living now the life you really want, a life you chose and created consciously and deliberately? Or did it just kind of happen?

Because despite what you may currently think, no one's life "just happens."

You created the life you live today just as every other person did. The problem is that you weren't consciously aware of the plan you were working to, the one that was given to you by your parents, teachers, and friends.

And because you weren't aware of it, you didn't really stop to consider whether it was the right plan for you.

Have you ever taken the time to think about where your model of the world comes from? That is the specific blueprint you follow in your life: your core beliefs, values, and the rules you give yourself that govern your entire life.

Have you taken time to figure out what you really wanted in life?

- The kind of person you wanted to become
- The kind of partner you wanted to have
- What your life purpose was
- What your real dreams and ambitions were

For 99% of people, the answer to that question is NO! They don't really want what *they* want, they want what they have been **PRECONDITIONED** to want.

- They want what their parents told them they should want.
- They want what their partners say they should want.
- They want what their friends think "everyone" should want.
- They want what their teachers taught them they should want.
- They want what society expects them to want.

As a young child, **you knew exactly what you wanted** and it didn't matter at all what other people thought. You never considered living by someone else's rules. Life was wide open. You knew you could be, do, or have anything.

But as you grew up you became progressively socialized – taught what you should do, what you should say, what you should think. You were taught society's rules, the path that you should follow to become society's definition of successful, and live what others defined as a good life.

What you really wanted, what really made you happy, slowly got buried under layers and layers of false programming and stifling social conditioning about the way things should be.

You also learned, most importantly, that you needed to take on these rules and these models and live by them *in order to be accepted and loved*.

Your model of the world, your vision of how things are supposed to be, is all prompted by the childhood realization that being loved is conditional, that you need to in some way conform in order to be accepted. As a result, we develop a set of rules to meet those conditions and be loved.

THE TWO CRITICAL QUESTIONS THAT DEFINE NEARLY EVERYONE'S LIVES

What forces could be strong enough to make us give up – or even forget – what we really want and do the bidding of others?

One of my two most important mentors is Stephen Hedger. Stephen is the top relationship coach in the UK and, in my opinion, the world. People like me go to Stephen when all else has failed. Having worked with hundreds of people both individually and as couples, he has a unique and unparalleled understanding of what drives people to take on damaging, self-defeating behaviors that have undermined and damaged themselves and their relationships.

During one of our conversations, he told me that there were two questions that defined nearly everyone's lives. They sat right at the very core of our psychology and ultimately drove our thoughts, choices, decisions, and actions.

These questions were:

1) Am I enough?

2) Will I be loved?

Each of us, at our very core, is driven by one of these two questions, sometimes both.

Our darkest fear, often hidden away, is that somehow, in some way, we are not enough or that we are in some way fundamentally unlovable.

Being "enough" and being loved are core, almost primal needs; fulfilling them causes you to override every other choice, consciously or unconsciously. And you can become unconsciously self-destructive in order to meet those needs above all others.

As a child, when your survival is dependent on others, those fears can be greatly heightened. So when approval, praise, or love is given as a reward for doing what you "should," or withheld as a punishment for not doing what you "should," you will do that to the point of self-destruction.

Repeat this pattern enough and you will forget <u>how to not do it</u>. Over time, it becomes your new default programming.

You stop focusing on what you want and instead focus on what makes you feel like you are enough or worthy of love as defined by an arbitrary set of rules and judged by an arbitrary set of people.

So now, in order to be accepted and loved, you start twisting your own model and blueprint to align it with those rules. Slowly, bit by bit over time, you stop being aware of what you really want and become increasingly aligned with that blueprint.

You end up completely bent out of shape, and if you're anything like most people, you have absolutely no idea what's happened – apart from the fact that life doesn't make sense and you don't feel good.

But how can you feel good when you're following someone else's plan for your life? When you've given up on your real dreams, your real passions, your real goals, your true values?

<u>When you've given up on being the real you</u>?

You feel bad because you are working harder and harder to achieve a dream that isn't even yours.

You're working really hard to live a life that doesn't align with your real values and your real identity.

You are striving to become a person who isn't aligned with their true passions, their true identity, their true values, and their true purpose.

Internal conflict is inevitable. And the biggest problem is that hardly anyone is even aware of this.

How can life make sense when meeting core foundational needs means working against your desires, dreams, goals, and aspirations? How can you be happy, confident, and successful when you're working against what you really want?

If you want to live a life that makes sense, the first step you've got to take is to stop following a blueprint you didn't even create.

The first step on that journey (which you've just taken) is to become aware that you are following someone else's blueprint, someone else's design for your life, and that you've lost touch with what you truly want.

There is incredible power in simply observing without judgment how your thoughts, actions, and choices all align with a model that you didn't choose. Now you can start to see where all the problems, the pain, the confusion, and the choices that didn't work for you ultimately came from.

UNDERSTANDING WHO YOU REALLY ARE

The second step to real and lasting change, to become the person you really want to be, and to create the life you really want to live, is to **shift your identity**, your sense of who you are.

The reason so many people fail to make lasting change in their life is because most personal development tackles the problem at the wrong level.

It focuses on changing your behavior, but it never shifts your identity.

The problem? That goes against the natural workings of our minds. Everything about who we are and how we operate in the world flows from how we see ourselves. The way we talk, our body language, the eye contact we make, the way we express what we think and feel, the level to which we stand up for ourselves, the confidence we have – these all stem from our self-perception.

If you see yourself as worthy and deserving, if you're proud of who you are and confident of your place in the world, then your behaviors, choices, and body language will align with that, naturally and without effort. It is easy, natural, and congruent. And it takes no effort whatsoever to sustain. You simply operate naturally at that level.

But if you see yourself as unworthy and undeserving, you can learn everything there is to know about body language, eye contact, how to be assertive, etc., and you may be able to put each element into practice – but the pieces won't align. Aligning the pieces will take enormous effort that will end up exhausting you, and you will ultimately slip back to your previous default state.

Except you won't just go back to where you were before. You'll likely feel worse.

You'll "believe" (because that's what all the books and courses tell you) that you've found all the answers but that they haven't worked for you. And so now, there's something even *more* fundamentally wrong with you than you thought before: because another book hasn't worked; another "answer" has failed to bring about the lasting, powerful change you wanted.

But none of that is true and it's the wrong process anyway.

The process of changing your identity might sound hard but it's actually nowhere near as difficult as it may appear.

Because confidence and success aren't about **changing away** from who you are.

They are about **changing back** to the person you <u>always were</u>.

Can you see the difference? Can you feel the difference?

One way says that you are fundamentally a flawed, damaged, broken human being who needs to move away from themselves in order to become well, decent, lovable, and successful.

The right way says that you are <u>***already***</u> all of the things you desire to be.

You have simply forgotten and buried that incredible, gifted, and naturally talented person under the weight of bad teaching, awful programming, and stifling social conditioning.

You see, all of these layers of conditioning and teaching became who you thought you were. It wasn't really who you were, just what you had been taught was who you were.

And at a very deep level you intuitively knew you were self-sabotaging, working against yourself, and acting in ways that you didn't like and weren't proud of.

So, you came to not like who you were. But in reality, the person you haven't liked, felt good about, or felt confident about being *is the identity that embodies all this bad teaching*.

Which isn't the real you.

Much of the teaching in this book is about doing exactly that: removing all the bullshit bad teaching and social conditioning that took you away from being who you really are. When you remove that bullshit and unblock the natural success and confidence mindset you were born with, your life will transform in a profound, lasting natural way.

Because you will just be YOU, probably for the first time since you were a child.

And that is why it will last.

THE ONE KEY MINDSET CHANGE FOR CONFIDENCE AND SUCCESS

In her brilliant book *Mindset*, Carol Dweck highlights one of the basic beliefs we hold about ourselves, and shows how this single mindset foundationally determines the degree to which we become the person we want to be and whether we accomplish the things we value.

There are two basic mindsets: a fixed mindset and a growth mindset.

SIDE NOTE

As you read this, your ego may try to persuade you that you have one mindset instead of the other, the one it thinks you "should" have. Observe your ego trying to do this and, for now, allow yourself not to judge. Just read and consider this section and allow yourself to find which mindset you have adopted in the past. No matter which mindset you may already have, learning this will help you – if you apply it. If you find you have a mindset that's held you back, then you should be delighted with yourself because you've just found a huge piece of the puzzle to help you get the life you want.

A fixed mindset assumes that your character, intelligence, talents, and abilities are set in stone – fixed things that are predetermined at birth. The fixed mindset believes that who you are and what you are capable of becoming can't be changed in any meaningful way.

Your life, achievements, confidence, and success are then simply reflections of the cards you were dealt at birth. What you achieve is just a way of proving, assessing, and measuring those pre-existing facts about who you are.

Someone with a growth mindset sees themselves and the world completely differently.

For those with a growth mindset, who you are and what you are capable of is not fixed or static. Your character, skills, and abilities are not carved in stone and something you just have to live with.

Instead, the hand you're dealt is simply *the starting point for your development*. Your skills, talents, intelligence, and character are all things that you can develop and cultivate through action, application, and experience. Although people are very different, everyone can change and grow.

The consequences of these different mindsets, of believing that your intelligence, personality, and who you can be is either predetermined or something to be developed is astonishing.

Your mindset profoundly impacts the way you lead your life and determines a great deal of your behavior. Far more importantly, however, is that it defines your relationship with success or failure, and as a result, defines your _**capacity**_ for happiness, confidence, and success.

Take a moment to look at the table below (based on the graphic by Nigel Holmes), and consider which mindset you have held in your life so far.

Fixed Mindset _Intelligence and ability are static_	TWO MINDSETS	Growth Mindset _Intelligence and ability can be developed_
Leads to a desire to look smart and therefore a tendency to......		Leads to a desire to learn and therefore a tendency to.......
...avoid challenges	**CHALLENGES**	...embrace challenges
...give up easily	**OBSTACLES**	...persist in the face of setbacks
...see effort as fruitless or worse	**EFFORT**	...see effort as the path to mastery
...ignore useful negative feedback	**CRITICISM**	...learn from criticism
...feel threatened by the success of others	**SUCCESS OF OTHERS**	...find lessons and inspiration in the success of others
As a result, they may plateau early and achieve less than their full potential	**RESULT**	As a result, they reach ever higher levels of achievement

Slow down as you do this. Remember this is just for your benefit. Don't worry about what you think you should be or beat yourself up for not being it. Just enjoy finding an answer.

One of the most powerful revelations from understanding these mindsets is how they drive your behaviors, your choices, and the paths you take; how they create the feelings you hold about yourself and how they help you or harm you on your journey to being who you want to be and creating the life you want to live.

People with fixed mindsets, for example, get consumed with the goal of proving themselves, of needing to use situations to confirm their underlying abilities. Carol Dweck describes a fixed mindset as, *"always trying to convince yourself and others that you have a royal flush when you're secretly worried it's a pair of tens."*

Fixed mindset people need approval and external validation as a means of reinforcing their internal sense of their fixed traits. Failure is therefore to be feared because it "reveals" the underlying fixed truth of who they are and so could shatter that person's identity and sense of value.

Conversely, people with a growth mindset are **driven to learn** rather than seek approval. They have a hunger to learn because they know that they will get better, stronger, and more powerful through experience and deliberate practice.

They may share the word failure with their fixed mindset peers but the emotional meaning attached to that word is entirely different. They don't emotionally experience failure as something they got wrong.

They see failure as a pure learning experience.

This means that instead of hiding their flaws or feeling ashamed about not being perfect, they shine a bright light on them and have a passion for learning how to overcome them. This creates a resilience that is astonishingly powerful and allows them not only to survive but actually thrive during their most challenging times.

Learning and, more importantly, living the growth mindset profoundly changes your experience of life. Instead of focusing on *appearing smart*, good, or talented, you instead switch your focus to actually *becoming smarter, better, and more talented*. As Carol Dweck says:

"When you enter a mindset, you enter a new world. In one world — the world of fixed traits — success is about proving you're smart or talented. Validating yourself. In the other — the world of changing qualities — it's about stretching yourself to learn something new. Developing yourself.

"In one world, failure is about having a setback. Getting a bad grade. Losing a tournament. Getting fired. Getting rejected. It means you're not smart or talented. In the other world, failure is about not growing. Not reaching for the things you value. It means you're not fulfilling your potential.

"In one world, effort is a bad thing. It, like failure, means you're not smart or talented. If you were, you wouldn't need effort. In the other world, effort is what makes you smart or talented."

If you identified that you have lived with a fixed mindset so far, be delighted because you've just uncovered one of the critical blocks to creating the confidence and success you desire. You have found the roadblock that's preventing your progress on your journey.

Understand that you have a choice, a choice you can make anytime you like (like right now!) to adopt the mindset shift that dissolves that roadblock in front of your eyes – the mindset that allows you to begin to access your true potential.

Don't let your ego make you feel bad about "the time you have wasted" or persuade you that you cannot change. This is your ego trying to keep you stuck and playing small. Drowning you in regret for the past, sabotaging you with the lie that it's too late for you.

Instead, all you need to do is recognize the truth that you have found an answer that helps you; that unlocks the talent and greatness that you know exists within you, lying dormant until you set it free.

You can set it free today.

THINGS TO CONSIDER

- Can you begin to see that you were born naturally confident and successful? That being confident and successful is your natural state? And that you've simply been taught a series of damaging, limiting, and sabotaging ways of thinking that have blocked this natural confidence and success mindset?

- Can you see that there's nothing wrong with you, the real you, that you're not broken and don't need fixing?

- Consider that the journey to confidence and success is not about changing away from who you are, but changing back to the real you, the person you really are underneath all the bad teaching and backwards thinking that blocks so many people's potential.

- Can you see that without understanding this crucial point, all books, courses, and therapy will end up making you feel worse about who you are rather than better? How they will take you away from your natural confidence and success instead of towards it?

- Consider: Whose blueprint for your life have you been following? Is it one you chose for yourself? Would you choose it again now or would you choose something different?

- Consider how behavior follows identity – not the other way around – and that when you see the truth about who you really are and the incredible talents, gifts, and joy you bring to the world, all of your behavior naturally starts to shift as a result.

- Consider whether up until now you have unconsciously lived with a fixed mindset. Consider if you want to continue with that fixed mindset or if you can see how choosing to have a growth mindset would help you unleash the incredible gifts within you. Consider if you want to make that change today and if there is any benefit to you in waiting. Don't judge, just consider.

CHAPTER 2

HOW TO WIN THE BATTLE FOR CONTROL OF YOUR MIND

> You have absolute control over just one thing: your thoughts. This divine gift is the sole means by which you may control your destiny. If you fail to control your mind you will control nothing else.
>
> NAPOLEON HILL

What if I told you that there was *one skill* that was the master key to everything you wanted in life?

That mastery of this skill virtually *guarantees* that you would become the person you want to be and live the life you want to live?

That if you learned, practiced, and then mastered this skill you would be able, on demand, to create success in whatever area of your life you desired, dissolve any self-limiting beliefs, and feel calm, confident, and clearheaded no matter the situation?

Now, just to reinforce this a little more, what if I now also told you that virtually every great teacher, every spiritual master through the ages has confirmed that this is indeed the secret to life?

For those of you that are not spiritual, what if I told you that Tim Ferriss calls this the "meta-skill," by which he means that learning this skill allows you to <u>access and improve all others</u>.

He says that after interviewing more than 200 world-class performers for his podcast, with guests ranging from celebrities and business titans to athletes and special forces commanders, that this one skill is **the single thing** that sets them apart from everyone else.

Would you be interested to know what it was?

More importantly, would you be interested enough to learn it, to apply it, and then to practice it _until you've become a master of it_?

I trust I now have your attention and you understand the importance of what's coming next.

The master skill is the ability to **control your mind**, to control and focus the thoughts that you think.

This might sound simple, but less than 1 in 100 people have mastered this skill.

The question to ask yourself is, are you in control of your mind or is your mind in control of you?

Can you calm your mind when you want to, can you choose the thoughts that you want to think? Or does your mind run on autopilot, serving you up unhelpful, negative thoughts about what might happen, all the things that could go wrong, the things that you should have done, that you should feel bad about, that you got wrong?

How often does your mind distract you away from the things that would help you live the life you want, **just when you are about to start making progress**?

Just when you're on the verge of making a positive change, suddenly you feel the need to check your phone, look at Instagram, text a friend, watch something on YouTube.

How many times have you tried to make a positive change in your life but somehow at every turn something happens to stall, block, undermine, or just generally sabotage your progress?

All of that happens because you have not yet mastered the foundational skill of controlling what happens in your mind.

WHY THOUGHT CONTROL MATTERS

Nothing happens without a thought.

Everything you have ever done or not done started with a thought in your mind; all the feelings you've ever felt; all the actions you ever took; all the choices you ever made; all the opportunities you took or turned down; all of it, the whole lot, started with the thoughts in your mind.

Your life today is a direct reflection of your thinking; the person you are, the work that you do, the place you live, your partner, your friends, the amount of money you have, and yes, your confidence all flow directly from your thoughts.

But the problem is that most people don't choose the thoughts they think, because they are not in control of their mind.

Their thoughts are random, chaotic, full of fear, doubt, and self-limiting illusions. So, who they become and what they achieve is a tiny fraction of their true potential.

Now consider for a moment what you have achieved in your life. It's probably quite a lot.

You've achieved all of that <u>despite the fact that you're not in control of your mind</u> and that your mind is full of doubts, worries, and fears.

Imagine if instead of the vast majority of your thoughts being out of control and negative, that they were instead, calm, controlled, and focused on giving you exactly what you needed to progress in life.

Imagine what you could achieve then. You've achieved incredible things against the odds. So, imagine what's possible when you *change the odds in your favor*.

If your dominant thoughts are confident, relaxed, happy, and certain of your success, then that is the blueprint for the life you are creating.

HOW TO CONTROL YOUR MIND

So how do you actually learn to control your mind? Well, the technique I'm about to give you is the simplest and most powerful tool for mastering control of your mind.

WARNING

This technique will do NOTHING for you if you do not actually use it. Just reading it won't do anything. Given everything you've just read about all the incredible people who say this skill lies behind their success, take a moment to consider whether it's worth trying, rather than just reading about and moving on. Don't be deceived by how simple this technique appears: its simplicity is what makes it so powerful. But, slow down so you don't use this simplicity to dismiss the power of what you're being taught here.

I was taught this technique by my friend and mentor Andy Shaw in his brilliant book, *Creating A Bug Free Mind*. This technique kept me calm, focused, and clearheaded in ways that blew me away during the white heat of a very difficult divorce battle.

Andy first showed me this technique in 2011. Despite knowing Andy and knowing that what he taught worked, I ignored his clear and unambiguous advice that this was the most important thing he would ever teach me.

It took another six years and my life falling apart for me to become just desperate enough to get out of my own way and actually apply the advice of a trusted expert and friend.

Andy told me that the key to controlling my mind was to simply hold 15 seconds of uninterrupted positive thought – to take one wonderful, happy memory and think about <u>that thought and nothing else</u> for just 15 seconds.

The first time I tried this technique was a few days after my ex-wife told me that our marriage was over and that we were getting divorced.

At the time, it felt as though my life was completely falling apart and I was filled with anxiety, tension, fear, pain, hurt, and anger. I could barely hold any thought for even half a second.

My mind kept spinning off to all kinds of horrible scenarios of what might happen; the bad choices I might have made in the past; the pain and upset my children were about to face; that I might only get to see my children every other weekend; that I was likely to lose my home.

All these thoughts closed in on me and I felt completely overwhelmed.

But I knew a very difficult divorce battle was coming and that if I didn't get out of this spiral, get my head clear, and get ready for what was to come, that the consequences would be severe – and that they would impact not just the rest of my life but also the lives of my daughters.

So, I was *just desperate enough* to do whatever it took.

So that day, I finished my meetings at work, left early, and went for a long walk to clear my head. I walked to one of my favorite places, a bench on the Southbank next to the river in London. I sat on the bench, gently closed my eyes and just allowed my positive thought to come into my mind.

The thought that worked for me was a video of my eldest daughter Lara. She was about two at the time and I had been away on business in Australia for about 10 days. I had missed her hugely and couldn't wait to get home to see her.

I had a stopover in Singapore for a couple of hours and was just relaxing when my then wife sent through a video of Lara talking into the camera when she told her that "Daddy is coming home tomorrow."

Her beautiful face completely lit up with happiness and excitement at the thought of me coming home and she just started singing "Happy Birthday" with all the pure joy in the world just pouring out of her. It wasn't my birthday, by the way, but it was just her way of expressing the excitement, happiness, and joy she felt in that moment.

I find it hard, even now, to describe how I felt when I watched that video for the first time. I cried when I first got the video on my phone in Singapore. The happiness, love, the emotion was incredible. That was the thought that I tried to focus on for just 15 seconds.

But when I started, I could barely hold that thought for even one second!

This was one of the happiest, most joyful things that had ever happened to me and my mind wouldn't even allow me one second's peace to focus and enjoy it.

I tried again and after a few more attempts I could get to around two seconds before the negative thoughts came flooding in.

I realized that I essentially had no control of my own mind *at all*; that my mind was being controlled by something other than my conscious instructions. And it wouldn't allow me any breathing space to calm down, take a breath, feel good, and just take a little respite from all the chaos going on in my life at that time.

Andy had told me that I had a little terrorist running my mind and here it was being shown to me as clear as anything.

I kept going and I was clear in my own mind that no matter what I wasn't shifting off that bench until I managed to hold my thought for 15 seconds.

In the end it took me two hours.

That's two hours of practicing the technique and doing nothing else. Over those two hours I went from being able to hold the thought for a second or two, to a few seconds, until eventually I managed the 15 seconds.

After those two hours, I felt calmer than I had in months, and especially so compared to the days since my marriage had ended. Instead of my mind being completely chaotic and negative, I had experienced some moments of peace and clarity.

I started walking home, enjoying the calm feeling I now had. Each time I started feeling out of control again, or my fears and anxieties flared up, I went back to the 15 seconds of positive thought. I repeated it over and over, all the way home. I didn't manage the full 15 seconds every time, but each time I tried I got a little better.

Instead of just reading the technique that Andy had showed me years before (and which I had ignored up until now), I finally applied it and found an answer, a building block to help me through the challenge I was facing and to help me start creating the life I desired.

Not only did I feel calmer, but just as Andy had told me would happen, answers, ideas, insights, and moments of inspiration started to happen. Problems that previously seemed completely insurmountable became… just situations to deal with.

With my mind calm, I had moments of clarity and inspiration that completely turned the tide of a very difficult situation in my favor.

I started to be able to detach and just observe the insanity of all the thoughts racing through my mind – all the fears, anxieties, and doomsday scenarios playing over and over in my mind became things happening "over there," things that I was <u>a witness to</u> rather than things that were <u>happening to me</u>.

I kept practicing this technique over and over, and eventually it became something I could use on demand. As soon as I felt my mind slipping out of control, I would use this technique and then instantly, I was back in control.

This technique is the single most important reason I have been able to rebuild my confidence, my sense of myself, and my life. It stopped me from tumbling down into very dark places and losing years of my life in the process.

It turned my process of recovering from the horrible situation I was in from decades to days.

THE PROCESS FOR REGAINING CONTROL OF YOUR MIND

So here's how you do this.

I want you to think of something from your past – the happiest memory you have. A thought, a memory that, more than any other, fills you up, makes you happy, and makes you feel great whenever you think of it.

Something that no matter what, no one could ever take away from you. Make sure this is one that feels right to you, not one you think you should pick. Make it one that genuinely makes you feel amazing.

What matters is that you have a really strong, positive emotional connection with that memory.

It could be a happy memory from your childhood, a moment of incredible joy or peace when you were on holiday, a view that took your breath away the first time you saw it, an incredible sunrise or sunset, a beautiful beach, the moment your child was born, a moment with a pet.

Remember, you don't have to justify your choice of memory to anyone else. This is only for you and for your benefit.

Now take that memory, gently close your eyes and allow yourself to become completely immersed in it. **Soak in it.**

Feel the feelings you had when you first experienced that wonderful moment. Remember the smells, the sounds you heard, how the air felt around you.

Make the memory as vivid and immersive as feels right. Experience that moment again; live it again.

Just rest in that wonderful perfect moment.

Now think that thought and nothing but that thought for 15 seconds.

Can you do it?

If you actually tried this then you almost certainly couldn't hold the thought for more than a few seconds at best.

Keep practicing until you can. Don't get frustrated if it doesn't happen straightaway. You're learning a new skill and breaking a habit that you have probably had for years. Instead, be grateful and delighted that you are taking the first and most important step towards creating the life that you desire.

Be excited that you are learning the most important skill that there is to learn and that mastering this skill will unlock everything you want in life.

Don't "try" when you do this, just calmly rest on the thought.

Give it a go now.

Did you do it? Or did you skip past it without trying?

If you didn't make an attempt, consider why you decided to skip this exercise, given everything you've been told about how important and foundational this skill is.

I can show you this technique; I can show you the incredible costs to your life for not mastering it, and the astonishing benefits of becoming the master of your mind. But in the end, only you can choose to apply it.

Nothing is more important than learning this skill. This is the first and most crucial step on your journey to becoming the person you want to be and living the life you want to live. Without regaining control of your mind, all of your efforts will ultimately fall short.

If I could go back in time and give myself just on piece of advice, it would be to master this one skill sooner.

Now when you "try" to do this and your mind starts dragging you off in all kinds of directions, just detach and observe the craziness going on in your mind. Without judging as good or bad, as that doesn't help you, observe how your mind jumps about from thought to thought, and how nearly all of those thoughts are fears, doubts, distractions, worries, things you forgot to do, and things you "really" should be doing right now instead of practicing this.

THE LITTLE TERRORIST BETWEEN YOUR EARS

If you've spent any time doing that exercise, you've just been introduced to your ego, the little terrorist that sits inside all of our minds.

Every time you got distracted, fearful, anxious, or doubted yourself while you were trying to do that exercise, it was your ego messing with you.

This is the negative voice in your head that you think *is you*, and that throws all kinds of negative, undermining, limiting, toxic, damaging thoughts and feelings at you all day long. Every time "you" say to yourself, "You're not good enough," "You can't do that," "Good things like that never happen to you," "You're not the kind of person that great things happen to," and a thousand other thoughts like those, it's not really you. It's your ego.

If you are not feeling confident, not living the life you want and being who you want to be, this is why. You have a little terrorist running your mind and fighting against you in a battle you didn't even know you were fighting.

Stop and think about what this means. If you're anything like I was at that time, then you are almost never in control of your mind. You may think you've been trying really hard to make the changes you want in your life and become the person you want to be but the real you hasn't been running the show.

And if you're not in control of your thoughts, then how can you be in control of your actions, your choices, and your behaviors?

Over the course of this book, I will show you many more ways that your ego sabotages your efforts to grow, to feel good, and to create the life you want. But right now, I want you to get introduced to your own ego.

When we're first born, we don't have an ego. And that is exactly why we are able to achieve so many incredible things in the first few years of our lives. From being helpless when we're first born, by the age of three we learn to smile, laugh, crawl, walk, run, jump, eat, and play, and we learn the basics of social interaction.

We do all of this in three short years because we don't have our ego getting in our way.

But from around that age we start to really get socially conditioned. Because we can now speak, interact, and understand what others are telling us, we start to take on board what we are told. And because at that age our brains are like incredible sponges soaking up masses of information, without filters to keep the good and remove the bad, we start the process of taking on thought patterns that harm us.

We start to get told the things we "can't do," instead of just getting on and doing things as we did in those first three years. We start to get told what people "like us" "should" be, do, and have.

And most importantly, we start to realize that love is conditional.

So, we quickly learn and adapt to what we have to be and not be in order to be loved. By accident or design, we learn a vision of how we are "supposed to be" and so we develop an identity and a set of rules to meet those conditions to be loved.

Before the age of about three, you hadn't really developed enough awareness to know what being loved meant; you simply did whatever you had to do to get your needs met.

But from around the age of three, you stop focusing on what you want and you start focusing on all the "shoulds" (should be, should do, should have, should look, should sound like, etc.) so you get the love and acceptance that lies at the very core of what we all need and want the most.

Over time and without you even realizing it, these shoulds become your identity, who you come to believe you are.

Soon enough, this way of behaving starts to crystalize into the patterns that you run in your life in response to all kinds of situations. They become your default way of thinking, so ingrained and normalized that you stop being aware that they are there.

And they are so incredibly powerful because they are anchored to that childhood need for love and acceptance, to what feels like your very survival.

Over time, countless interactions with parents, friends, partners, social media, and teachers all add further layers onto this, until you become a full-fledged socially conditioned adult.

By now, 99% of people are so wrapped up in so many layers of social conditioning, muddled thinking, limiting beliefs, doubts, fears, concerns, and perceived lack of worthiness that they become almost entirely disconnected from their real selves.

But not fully disconnected.

The real you is still there. And it knows the truth.

It knows what you are truly capable of.

It knows that you are worthy of everything great that life has to offer.

It knows that the bullshit social conditioning is pure lies that holds you back and weighs you down.

It still serves you up dreams that it knows you can achieve.

But your ego fights against those dreams, against the real you rebelling within.

The real you fights back against the tyranny of your ego serving negative propaganda every time you try to grow, become more, and fulfill your true potential.

And so, you have massive internal conflict and pain. This is what my friend Richard Wilkins calls the civil war between your ears.

The real you knows your potential is essentially unlimited, just like when you were first born. It knows that only a bunch of crap thinking stands between you and all you desire.

The pain and regret that you feel exists because deep down you know you can, you know you are worthy, you know you are good enough.

If you knew, and I mean really knew, that your dreams were impossible, there wouldn't be any pain. That pain only exists because those dreams are not only possible, but actually easily attainable by the real you.

But your ego exists to keep you safe, to keep you "loved" and "accepted." So, it does whatever the hell it needs to do to stop all progress dead in its tracks. It knows you have survived your life so far, and the past is its only frame of reference. Its greatest fear is you doing something new. It knows if you don't do anything new then it will keep you safe.

So, every attempt to create something better in your life is met with immediate and serious resistance. It tells you nasty things will happen to you if you take a chance; that you're being responsible to worry about everything that could go wrong instead of being carefree and looking at all the amazing possibilities for your life like you did when you were a young child (remember how much you achieved during that time...).

That if you become confident, then you're a fake; that no one will like you; that they will stop liking and accepting you. After all, you've already been told all the dangers and fears and bad stuff that can happen if you attempt something great; if you start that business, you could lose your home; if you approach that hot girl/guy, they could reject you and that would be just too much.

But the biggest problem is that most people think that voice is them. Since about the age of three, you've been in a battle for control of your mind that you didn't even know you were fighting.

I want you to slow down for a moment because the next bit I'm about to tell you is really important.

All those bad feelings you have had about yourself, all those times you've felt crap about who are, they aren't your feelings about you, the real you.

They're your feelings about your ego.

Your bad feelings are about the little terrorist between your ears who has spent most of your life kicking the shit out of you for every attempt to do something good, to try things, to grow. Your ego is the very worst version of all the bad stuff you ever got taught.

Is it any surprise you don't have a lot of positive feelings about that "person"?

Whereas when you slow down and take a moment to remember the real you who's still there inside – kind, decent, loving, excited about the world, adventurous, full of possibility and potential – then your feelings are very different.

Take this slowly because right now your ego will be going into overdrive, taking all kinds of shots at what's written here, desperately looking for distractions – compelling you *to check your social media, listen to music, do those household chores, make that phone call, send that email.*

All of these distractions are your ego trying to take you away from this, because it knows when you realize the truth that it's losing its power over you.

Your ego has developed and grown out of control because you didn't know it even existed and because you haven't been taught how to control your thoughts. With your ego in charge you have muddled, destructive, limiting thoughts running your mind.

When you learn to control your mind and quiet your ego, the real you is suddenly in charge once again. Then you can start to create a life that makes sense for you.

And by realizing that your ego isn't the real you, you can start to reconnect with who you really are – the all-powerful real you – and with what you really want. You can begin being free of all that stifling social conditioning.

Here's the second really important thing I'm going to tell you in this section. So again, slow down and take a moment to consider this.

Putting the real you back in charge isn't as difficult as you might think. You already do this; you are already confident in areas of your life right now.

Maybe you're great at your job, great in relationships, a great parent, great at sports, great at computer games, great at singing, dancing, making friends, etc.

In those areas of your life where you are already doing well, you have already mastered this; you may simply not have realized that you did. And that is true of anyone who has ever mastered anything.

They (you) found a way, by accident or design, to get past the traps and blocks their (your) ego placed in their (your) path. They (you) silenced the doubts, the negative thinking, the limiting beliefs, the fears, and the shoulds, and simply just did whatever was necessary to get to the next step.

Do you see? You already know this way of thinking in specific areas of your life. All you now have to do is learn to apply that <u>across all areas of your life</u>.

The key to winning the battle with your ego is to not fight it, but instead relax and observe the madness. As counterintuitive as it may sound, the more you fight and resist your ego the more power you give it.

But if you relax and simply observe the craziness it throws at you all day long, its power simply falls away. You don't need it to stop, but simply observing the insanity, simply looking at whether all those thoughts help you or keep you stuck dissolves all of its power.

One last thing, and I really cannot emphasize this enough. Becoming aware of your ego and its tricks to keep you stuck, and learning to control your thoughts are the foundational skills you **must acquire** to become who you want to be and create the life you want to live.

Through the rest of this book, I will bring you back to this point many times. It is only through mind control that you can use the full focus of your mind's power in the right way, which helps you, instead of the wrong way, which sabotages you.

When I repeat this message, observe your ego trying to get you irritated with my repetition, trying to distract you, or simply trying to get you to not practice the skill because you "already know it."

ULTIMATE THOUGHT CONTROL – THE POWER OF "NO MIND"

After you've managed to bring in the 15 seconds of positive thought, the next stage is what Andy calls "No Mind." This is when you literally think of nothing – no thoughts at all. It is complete presence, awareness, calmness, and serenity.

When I bring in No Mind, all my thoughts quiet, and then simply stop. It is a lovely, calm, peaceful feeling that gently washes over me. I feel like I am in the world and separate at the same time.

I often start off by imagining myself gently drifting down in a beautiful crystal clear blue sea. As I lie resting under the water, there is silence, peace, and I feel completely calm. I am aware of what's around me but cut off at the same time. Even if there was a storm above the water, underneath on the sea bed where I am it is completely peaceful. I mentally lie there resting, just relaxing into the feeling of my mind completely still, completely open, completely serene.

I stay in this state for as long as feels right to me. Sometimes it's only thirty seconds but often it's a couple of minutes.

Afterwards I feel clear and refreshed with my mind still and ready for whatever I want or need to deal with next. I feel full of energy, vibrant, and completely clear-minded. All the noise, all the chatter, all the chaos of the world is still going on but I emerge calm and primed. The chaos is "over there" and doesn't affect me at all.

When you are ready to allow this to happen, don't force it. Just relax into the feeling and silence your mind. The first times you do this its best to be somewhere very quiet and peaceful where you won't be disturbed. You don't want any external distractions.

When you bring in No Mind, see how long you can hold it for. You don't need to hold this for long. You'll be amazed at the changes inside your mind and your feelings by doing this for even a short time.

My advice is that you return to this chapter and this exercise again and again. I'm repeating and emphasizing this very deliberately. This is the most important thing you can do.

This simple exercise will transform your experience and your results in everything in life.

It really is the master skill of all skills.

Remember that the state you're in most often becomes your default setting.

The more you do this, the more you shift your default state from one of being out of control to one of being in complete control. This is retraining your default setting.

What this means is that by practicing regaining control of your mind and becoming calm, happy, and grateful, this becomes your default state, the state you are in all the time, pretty much no matter what.

And this is what we want to focus on.

Then, over time, that becomes your new normal, your new natural – your default setting that you naturally reset to no matter what.

It is the foundation to certain confidence, certain success in whatever area of life is important to you.

One mentor told me that things are hard the first few times you do them because you're creating new neural pathways. The first time is like walking through thick jungle with a machete, hacking through the branches and leaves. After a few times you've cleared a bit of a path and it is a little easier. After a hundred times you have a pretty good path. After ten thousand times you have a six-lane highway and there is only one way your thoughts will go after that.

This is what we're doing here. We're shifting things around in your mind to make it easier for you to be in control, calm, happy, and confident as your default state.

Don't worry if you haven't been able to do this yet. I didn't get it the first time. **But I did keep practicing until I did and that was the turning point.**

So do yourself a massive favor, go and take some time right now and keep practicing this until you get it.

As you get better at it, try it in more contexts and situations. When you're walking, when you're getting your coffee, when you're listening to music. Keep going until there is no situation where you cannot calm your mind and control your thoughts.

If you took one day out just to practice this one skill, you would see changes that would take your breath away. Andy told me to do this and I ignored it for over two years, until I was just desperate enough.

Once you've regained control of your mind, you've just accomplished the first step in becoming unstoppable and having indestructible confidence.

Let's now move on to setting more of the foundation for your unstoppable mindset.

THINGS TO CONSIDER

- Do you control your mind or does it control you? Slow down and consider this; don't answer straightaway. Look to your feelings for the answer.

- Consider: How much better would your life be if you had the power to only think the thoughts that helped you instead of thoughts that harm you?

- Consider: Have you brought in the 15 seconds of positive thought yet? Do you know, really know, that this is the foundational skill for all success?

- Are you now aware of your ego? Are you now aware that you have been in a battle for control of your mind and didn't even realize it?

- Consider that all the bad feelings you have had about yourself aren't feelings about the real you, but about your ego. Can you see how that changes the way you understand who you really are?

- Can you see how your ego has sabotaged your efforts to create the life you want to live and to become the person you want to be?

- Can you see how the battle for control of your mind between the real you and your ego leads to what my friend Richard Wilkins calls the civil war in your mind?

CHAPTER 3

BECOMING UNSTOPPABLE: THE MINDSET OF THE 1%

> **Whether you think you can or you can't you're right.**
>
> HENRY FORD

The way the 1% think and live is completely different from the other 99%. In fact, the differences are so profound that most people think the 1% are simply exceptional – that they are one-offs, gifted, lucky, or just wired differently from everyone else.

But those differences aren't simply some genetic quirk. The 1% aren't a different species. It is simply that the 1% have either **relearned** or **never lost** the natural confidence and success mindset that we are all born with.

Yes, that includes you too.

The 1% have what the world sees as a different operating system but is in fact the natural, all-powerful operating system you were born with too. The difference is that most people's operating system has been corrupted with all kinds of bugs and viruses – the bad teaching, the muddled backwards thinking, false assumptions, fears, doubts, and stifling social conditioning that so many people suffer with.

The good news is that you can uncorrupt your operating system and return your mind to its natural, confident, successful state. It is a process. And that means that anyone that follows the right process will get the result. Including you.

As Michael Gerber says, "Process permits ordinary people to achieve extraordinary results predictably." That's what's going to happen for you if you read, reread, and then most importantly _apply the lessons_ in this book. It's how you get repatterned back to your natural, all-powerful state.

But this change isn't hard work.

In fact, this will be some of the most exciting, enjoyable, liberating "work" you will ever do. As each change happens, you will see exciting, wonderful changes happen in your life. You will feel lighter and freer as you let go of each piece of baggage weighing you down that you hadn't even realized you were carrying.

You know that feeling when you've been carrying something heavy for a long time and you suddenly put it down? You not only have the relief of not carrying the heavy load but you feel lighter than you did before. That's the process we're doing together.

You're about to go through some wonderful, incredible changes. I'm excited for you. I'm even a little bit envious because I know just how incredible the journey is.

But first I want to give you an insight, a little guided tour of the mindset of the 1% to show you just how different it is from the way that most people think and to show you the mindset you will (re)create for yourself.

As you go through this section, take a few moments to imagine, to daydream about living with this new mind state. I want you to enjoy – now – the feeling of the mind state you will be creating.

We'll get into the details of this mindset and exactly how to create it later in the book. Right now, just relax and enjoy seeing how the 1%

think and how you too will think shortly. As you read through, consider *how little effort* each of these mindset traits dedicates to trying to be confident.

As I laid out at the start of this book, true lasting confidence must be created **without direct effort**. Confidence doesn't happen through trying to be confident, but from applying accurate, natural thinking to yourself and to your life.

STEP 1: SELF-KNOWING

The difference between great people and everyone else is that great people create their lives actively, while everyone else is created by their lives, passively waiting to see where life takes them next.

– MICHAEL GERBER

Do you know who you are?

That's one of those questions that most people answer without thought. They immediately think, "Yes, of course I know who I am" which means that they almost certainly don't know who they are.

So, before you jump in and answer, take a moment to consider this.

Do you know what you stand for, what your values are, what matters the most to you? Could you write it down now if I asked you to?

What are you willing to go into battle for? And just as importantly, do you know what doesn't matter to you?

Do you know what you won't tolerate in your life and must be eliminated, what you will stand against, even if it causes confrontation and makes you unpopular?

The answers to these questions are the building blocks of your identity. They create your self-perception and give it structure and integrity.

Your values set the framework for your life. They set the lens for how you see the world and the events that happen. They define the set of choices you decide are open to you and which ones are not.

If you don't know who you are and what you value, and most importantly, if you don't live those values, then by default, you simply fall into line with what feels easiest in the moment.

You become like a bottle, passively floating in the ocean, going wherever the prevailing current takes you.

How can you feel good about who you are if you don't know who you are?

How can you stand up for something if you don't really know what you want to stand up for?

How can you have self-esteem without a sense of integrity, an integrity that can only exist with a strong foundation of values?

The 1% know *exactly* who they are. In most cases, they actively designed who they wanted to become and <u>created themselves on purpose</u>.

They may have written this down or simply daydreamed about it in detail, but however it happened, they have a crystal clear vision of the best version of themselves. And they actively work towards that vision every day. Because they know that design and are proud of it, they know and like themselves by default.

They know and like the decisions they make, the behaviors they adopt, and the life they lead in alignment and integrity with that vision of the very best version of themselves.

They know their purpose in life and they work on it, without it feeling like work. They are inspired by what they do. Their lives are filled with purpose and meaning, but a purpose and meaning that they crafted so that it makes sense to them.

Nothing and no one could cause them to drift because they are too excited, too inspired by their journey. Their compass cannot drift from its magnetic north because the pull and excitement of their purpose and vision means that going anywhere else would be "less" than where they're headed.

Standing up for themselves and others is easy, because to not do it is to compromise that vision that they love.

Decisions are clear and generally easy. Each decision either helps them on their journey or slows them down. They have no interest in anything that doesn't help them become the person they want to be and create the life they want to live.

If you want to start to figure out your values, the simplest way is to simply consider what's really important to you and, just as importantly, what isn't.

A great place to start is to look at the six basic universal needs that drive all human behavior. This was formulated by the brilliant Tony Robbins and you can find the original article here: https://www.entrepreneur.com/article/240441.

We all have these six needs, but how we value and prioritize those needs determines what really drives each of us.

Need 1: Certainty/Comfort

The first human need is for certainty. At its core this is our survival mechanism. This is really about our need to feel in control and to know what's coming next so we feel safe. It's the need for basic comfort, the need to avoid or minimize pain and stress. How important this need is to you will define your appetite to take risks in life. It may vary between different aspects of your life such as your relationship or work. The more you need certainty in a given area, the less risks you are willing to take.

Need 2: Uncertainty/Variety

If life was fully, 100% certain and predictable we'd all be utterly bored. Everyone needs some excitement, some energy in their lives which comes from having a degree of uncertainty. The question is how much you value this excitement and variety and how much of it you want compared to your desired level of certainty.

Need 3: Significance

A great way to understand anyone's behavior is to understand where they get their significance from. We all need to feel important, special, and needed. But people activate their significance in a whole variety of ways – some healthy, some not. For example, some get it through having money (or by being frugal), some through their physical appearance, and some through being popular and famous, through the number of social media followers they have.

Some people equally get it by having bigger problems or by being more of a victim than anyone else.

But underlying all is the need to be seen, to be recognized, and to matter.

Need 4: Love and Connection

Another core need is love and connection. We all need to feel like we belong, and the highest form of belonging is to love and be loved for exactly who you are. The more conditionally we feel we are loved or the more conditionally we give love, the more or less fulfilled we will feel. This doesn't have to be intimate love, although it commonly is. Many people also get this sense of love and connection through friendship, spirituality, or even through animals and nature.

Need 5: Growth

Deep in our core is a drive for growth: to become the very best version of ourselves in whatever way we define it; to become the person we daydream about being; to experience creating and living the life we want to live. This is the highest form of self-expression, of being authentic and all of who we are.

Need 6: Contribution

We all want to feel like we're part of something bigger than ourselves, that we are making a difference, putting our dent in the universe. Whether it's through small acts of honor and kindness or making your work about something you completely believe in, that sense of contributing to those around you and the wider world matters. Life is about creating meaning.

And meaning does not come from what you get, it comes from what you give.

While you get pleasure from what you get, ultimately, it's who you become and what you contribute (the meaning of your life) that will make you happy long term.

Do you want to get a sense of your driving force and learn which need matters to you most? Tony Robbins has a short quiz to help you find out which you can access here: *https://core.tonyrobbins.com/driving-force-6/*

STEP 2: SELF-ACCEPTANCE

How much do you change of yourself to fit in? Do you become a social chameleon, always adjusting aspects of what you say, what you think, and how you act in order to be accepted and liked?

If you answered straightaway, it was your ego talking, not the real you. Instead, consider this slowly as it's only for your benefit.

Most people do this. They bend themselves out of shape, a little or a lot, in order to be accepted.

And in doing so they miss the obvious point that if they simply *accepted themselves* as they are, there would be no need to constantly become someone different in every circumstance or environment.

This behavior and, more importantly, the mindset behind it says, "I'm not enough as I am." I won't be liked or loved for simply being who I am, so to survive I must pretend to be something I'm not.

So many mistakenly believe that **being someone else means being something better**. And this toxic and entirely inaccurate belief eats away at your self-worth until eventually there's nothing left.

You can't like who you are if who you are constantly changes. Where's your core?

It's one of the reasons I hate the "fake it till you make it" approach that so many people advocate. You're still faking it and you still know you're faking it.

It's way, way, way, better to simply realize the truth – the truth that the 1% never lost – and that is that the most empowering belief is also the most accurate.

You are enough, you always were, and you always will be.

You have simply been taught bad thinking and a whole host of limiting beliefs that caused you to understand otherwise.

You have no need to fake anything.

Simply being fully you, with love and respect is the most powerful, attractive, and life-changing thing you can do.

Then, instead of bending yourself out of shape to fit in, the world will adjust to fit in with you.

The 1% have genuinely no need for acceptance or validation from others; they know and accept fully to their very core exactly who they are. Their self-acceptance carries vastly more weight and value than an opinion from anyone else: good, bad, or indifferent.

They travel through life with a calm, peaceful confidence, certain of who they are and their value in the world. They don't fear the opinion or any lack of acceptance from others. They are already filled to the brim with their internal acceptance.

The problem is that so many people focus on being *liked* rather than being *respected*.

If you focus on being liked, then you are looking at **how you need to change yourself in order to get approval** from others.

This is muddled, self-sabotaging thinking.

It means you are willing to compromise who you are and what you stand for so that others will accept you.

You lose your core, your essence. And you cannot live life on your terms because your starting point is to live life on the terms that others have set for you.

Instead, if you focus on being respected, you are focused on your values, your principles, and your purpose.

You become a person of unshakable integrity, and you do the right thing even if that choice is unpopular.

You remain true to yourself which means that even those who don't "like" you respect you.

And then, ironically, you become accepted for who you are.

STEP 3: SELF-RESPECT

How much are you on your own side?

How much do you expect people to treat you well, with integrity and respect?

How much do you make time for the things that are important to you and your life?

Most people unconsciously allow the things that matter the most – their conscious, active self-respect, their goals and dreams, their needs and priorities – to fall by the wayside.

In the busyness of life, the things that fill them up get pushed down their priority list, waiting for "one day" when they have time.

All too often, they unconsciously accept disrespectful, careless, thoughtless behavior that leaves them feeling devalued.

They fall into the trap of remaining passive in these situations, waiting and looking for others to be their advocate, for others to stand up for them.

But unless **you show that you matter**, that your needs matter, and that you will only accept respectful behavior, why would you expect others to?

Unless you show that you appreciate your inherent value and actively set the standard for how others should behave towards you, how can you expect others to meet that standard <u>instead of making one up for themselves</u>?

This isn't being selfish and I'm not suggesting you ignore or casually disregard the needs of others.

I am absolutely saying that unless you consciously choose to make yourself and your life a priority, you are unconsciously choosing for it not to be.

You can't outsource that to someone else.

You have to be the leader in your life; you have to set the standard.

STEP 4: SELF-LOVE

Ever loved someone so much you would do anything for them? Well make that someone yourself.

– HARVEY SPECTRE

Would you feel comfortable telling people that you love yourself?

Would you feel proud to tell the world that you genuinely and deeply love **you**, in the same way that you would be proud to say that you love your partner, your family, your children, or *your dog*?

We are taught that completely and unconditionally loving another is something to aspire to – almost the pinnacle of human experience.

Yet we are taught that feeling exactly the same way about yourself is not just unworthy, but vain, arrogant, and conceited.

Somehow, it's OK to focus on the good and accept the flaws in others and love them without condition. But to offer the same love to yourself makes you vain and narcissistic.

Then most self-help books come along and tell you to love yourself.

Consider how insane this is for a moment.

So many people spend their whole lives striving to feel better about themselves and yet they have been taught that this very act of liking and loving themselves is something "bad."

The wickedness and stupidity of this teaching really is something else.

Can you imagine saying to a precious young child that it's wrong for them to like who they are? That it's not OK for them to feel that they are amazing, beautiful, wonderful, and incredible just as they are?

Yet how many people have told themselves precisely this lie thousands of times over?

As a result, they create a negative spiral in their own minds that makes their failure inevitable.

Because every attempt to feel better is blocked by the entirely false view that self-love equals conceit. How can you aspire to something you've been taught is bad and that you associate with all things negative?

Their egos confuse self-loathing with humility, make finding fault with themselves a virtue.

The 1% never got successfully programmed with this lie. They are entirely comfortable not only with loving themselves but with having a deep, unconditional love for themselves as their highest aspiration.

They know that loving themselves means exactly what it says and nothing more. It is a simple, kind, non-judgmental caring for yourself.

They know that just because most of the world also thinks it means vanity and arrogance doesn't make it true.

STEP 5: SELF-FORGIVENESS

Self-compassion is simply giving the same kindness to ourselves that we would give to others.

– CHRISTOPHER GERMER

Are you a kind and decent person?

Are you sure?

The reason I emphasize this question is because many people are far quicker to forgive others than themselves.

Most of the world aspires to compassion and forgiveness for the people around them. It is almost a defining characteristic of being a "good" person. Yet 99% of people don't apply anything like that standard to themselves.

Without seeing the obvious contradiction, they believe that being super hard on themselves and not forgiving themselves for their mistakes is noble.

Stop and ask yourself why you feel you don't deserve the same compassion and forgiveness you offer others.

Just as you cannot truly love another unless you truly love yourself, you cannot be a truly kind, compassionate, and forgiving person if you are unkind and lack compassion for yourself.

A very wise mentor of mine, Richard Wilkins, once asked me if I used my past as a library or a home.

What he meant by that was whether I used my past to learn the lessons I needed to live my best life or whether I lived in my past, stuck there filled with regrets.

That question had a profound impact on me.

Previously, my past had been a source of pain and regret. I didn't let go of the pain and so it defined my present and future, as well as my past.

Until you learn to forgive yourself, until you <u>unlearn the lie</u> that it's noble to beat yourself up for your human failings, you will remain anchored down with pain and baggage that has no benefit for you, for those you may have hurt, or for those you love. **For anyone.** In fact, it simply causes more pain in the present and so you end up creating more reasons to feel bad.

The 1% let go of their mistakes. They forgive themselves for whatever they may have done wrong because they know there is no benefit in doing anything else, in the same way that a young child (who has not yet been taught this terrible, awful programming) doesn't hang on to the past and so doesn't mess up their present.

STEP 6: SELF-EXPRESSION

Whenever you find yourself on the side of the majority, it is time to pause and reflect.

- MARK TWAIN

How much do you hold yourself back? How often do you shade your true thoughts and feelings so you don't upset others?

And how often do you sacrifice your opinions to not go against herd mentality, the majority opinion that becomes accepted wisdom, which is usually anything but wise?

Expressing fully who you are is your natural state. It means speaking with your authentic voice, stating your truth, not holding anything back out of fear of upsetting others or conventional, established thinking.

It means saying what you feel needs to be said, even when others don't want to hear it or when it may cause conflict.

It means giving the fullest expression of your talents to yourself, to those around you, and to the wider world.

You should express yourself with kindness, integrity, and respect because expressing who you are doesn't require you to silence others.

But don't hold back on yourself.

The 1% speak their truth and express their talents fully and without fear. Holding back makes no sense to them at all. In the same way as a young child just is, just does, and just expresses, so too do the 1%. They simply did not lose this natural mindset.

STEP 7: FEARLESS AUTHENTICITY

Authenticity is the daily practice of letting go of who we think we're supposed to be and embracing who we are.

– BRENÉ BROWN

You know that person you dream of being? The one you don't tell many people about? The person who accomplishes the dreams you have? Who says "FUCK YES!" to situations and opportunities your fears cause you to shy away from?

The one who is vibrant and full of energy, passion, and purpose?

Well say hello to the real you, the **authentic** you. It was and always has been the real you. As my friend Richard Wilkins says, "You are really a superhero pretending to be an ordinary person."

That's not some hokey bullshit. It's the truth.

It's just the truth you don't allow yourself to believe, but that doesn't make it any less true.

The greatest freedom in life is being completely, fearlessly, and unapologetically authentic.

You drop all the baggage; you throw off all the shackles and lose all the pretense. You no longer need to act or pretend, to second-guess yourself or what you "should" think, say, do, or be. You no longer need to hide anything about yourself from anyone.

It is complete and total acceptance and expression of who you are.

The 1% live this way by default. And the power it gives them is astonishing.

No more time, energy, and focus are wasted on building a façade, a patchwork life made up of all the things you are supposed to be, do, and have.

They don't need to waste any time proving themselves and their "worth" according to a false and arbitrary standard.

They are simply calm and still inside, at peace, and just being who they are – which requires no effort at all.

And so, they are free to make choices that make sense for them instead of for someone or something else.

They choose the rules. They choose the "shoulds" that make sense for them, not the ones that society has deemed to be right, yet cause untold misery for so many.

They readily and freely say "No" to the things that don't work for them and don't make sense to them.

And so, all their energy and focus are directed into being who they really are, instead of who society thinks they should be. They are then free to live life on their own terms.

THINGS TO CONSIDER

- Consider that the 1% who live life on their terms are not born differently from everyone else. It is simply that they have either **relearned** or **never lost** the natural confidence and success mindset that we are all born with.

- Consider that you were also born with the confidence and success mindset of the 1%. And you still have it. It's simply hidden under some layers of bad thinking and limiting programming that you, like 99% of the world, were taught.

- Consider that returning to this state is a process, which means that anyone who does the right steps in the right order will get the results. **Including you.**

- Consider: Do you truly know who you are? Don't answer right away, just consider.

- Consider: How can you feel good about who you are if you don't know who you are?

- Consider: Do you love, respect, accept, and forgive yourself easily? Each of these are core building blocks in your journey to recreating your natural confidence and success mindset. You don't need to try to do any of them. You simply need to stop tripping yourself up with the bad thinking that holds 99% back. Then these will all flow naturally.

FREE GIFT # 1 – BONUS LESSON: "HOW TO MASTER YOUR MIND"

If you'd like to go deep into learning how to master your mind – the "meta skill" that unlocks all others – go to **www. unstoppableselfconfidence.com/confidence-on-demand** and watch the first video in the free program where I share the steps I go through with my private clients to help create a calm, clear focussed mind no matter what life throws at them. I've also created some free cheat sheets to help you become the master of your mind faster. It's absolutely free. Enjoy.

02

HOW TO REMOVE THE BAD PROGRAMMING THAT'S HOLDING YOU BACK

CHAPTER 4

UNDERSTANDING YOUR TRUE POTENTIAL

Someone once told me the definition of hell: on your last day on earth, the person you became will meet the person you could have become.

ANONYMOUS

Did you know that less than 1% of people *ever* get to truly live the life they dream of?

Stop and think about that for a second.

Despite years of education, everything our teachers, parents, friends, and siblings taught us, all the books we've read, and all the courses we've done, **hardly anyone** achieves the goals, the dreams, the desires they have in life.

Yet somehow, despite being exposed to the same education and influences, the 1% do go on to achieve everything they want in life. So, it's demonstrably possible.

Does this mean that they are lucky, special, or gifted, that they are different from everyone else?

No. It simply means that they *failed to fail*.

Let me explain what I mean by that. We assume, without thought, that the purpose of the traditional education system is to teach us what we need to succeed in life. And we equally assume that the parenting, advice, and support we are given by our family, friends, and wider society is there to help us succeed.

And therefore, if we don't succeed, *we* must be the problem.

But what if that isn't true? What if the traditional system of education not only doesn't give you what you need to succeed but actually gives you (by accident or design) *what you need to fail*?

What if most of the advice you've been given by your parents, teachers, and friends, is the perfect system for not getting what you want in life, even if pretty much everyone thinks the opposite? And they think that way because they were also taught the same failing ways to think, act, and live.

Remember that the truth is the truth even if no one believes it and a lie is a lie even if everyone believes it.

HOW THE TRADITIONAL EDUCATION SYSTEM SETS YOU UP TO FAIL

A short history lesson will show you how and why the traditional education system sets you up to fail.

The education system that most countries still use is the Prussian education system. It originated in the eighteenth century and had very specific aims and objectives. (Take a moment to consider how many other things from the eighteenth century you still use today.)

The purpose of "education" was to create a useful generic worker, readily replaceable and dispensable. Students were taught only the most basic skills – enough to make them useful. The focus was on teaching obedience and uniformity. Originally, most pupils were boys as they would be the ones fighting any wars at the time.

This is why so many schools get pupils to stand when a teacher enters a room; why teachers were called by their formal names; why pupils often have to wear school uniforms; why classrooms often have regimented lines of desks; why pupils must raise their hands to speak; why questioning a teacher's decisions is frowned upon; why there is a school bell; and why pupils must stand in lines.

The curriculum consisted of learning by rote (memorizing) – reading, writing, and numeracy – and again, taught just enough basic information to be able to complete a simple task.

Tests were administered not to measure true understanding but the ability to memorize information and follow instructions – just like orders on a military mission.

Good students (those who society labels as high achievers) were those who memorize and follow instructions (i.e., obey orders) well. Those who rebel, who refuse to conform, who question, and who aren't interested in memorizing information for the sake of passing a test, were given bad grades and labelled as problem children.

Questioning, individuality, and creativity were all actively discouraged. Speaking up, expressing independent thought, and going against "the way things should be done" was not only frowned upon but actively punished.

The Prussian system was about creating obedient soldiers and workers who knew and understood *just enough* to serve a purpose, **but nothing more**. More knowledge was dangerous because that meant you might start doing something unhelpful like thinking for yourself!

This is a system designed to remove, stifle, and crush individuality, independent thought, and creativity, and to remove any sense that what you want or need matters. It is purposefully designed to condition and program blind, unquestioning obedience, and downgrading of the self to serve a bigger whole.

This is the system that was almost certainly used to educate you, your parents, your grandparents, your friends, your teachers (and their parents and grandparents). They were all taught the same failing programming. And so, the teaching and advice they give you is generally based on that same failed method of "learning."

I'm explaining this because I want you to understand that what you've achieved in your life so far has happened *in spite* of you being completely immersed in this tsunami of bad teaching.

So rather than beating yourself up for how little you think you've achieved, you've actually managed to achieve an incredible amount despite being taught a near perfect system *for failing at almost everything* that matters to you.

So, this is why I say that the 1% are simply the failures of the traditional education system. They live the life they want, and on their terms, because they failed (by accident or design) to take on board all the terrible, awful, wicked programming that seeks to turn you into a mindless automaton; to never reach for more than you're told is OK; to never question; to erase any sense that your needs and desires are important; to subvert your thinking, your will, and your decision-making to some "higher power."

Think of how much you achieved in the first few years of your life before you got caught by this teaching system. You learned to smile, laugh, crawl, walk, run, jump, communicate, play, and to socially interact with others. And you did all of that in the first few years of your life.

Without "being taught" any of it.

Your "education" gave you a set of limits instead of a world of possibilities. For example, according to research the average child is told "No" an astonishing 400 times per day! You were progressively told more and more things that you couldn't, mustn't, and shouldn't do. The more you progressed through the system, what you came to see as possible for your life became progressively smaller and narrower.

What's worse is that the more you "succeeded" in the traditional system, the more you were actually setting yourself up for failure later in life.

You were educated in limits not possibilities. You were educated in what you shouldn't do rather than what you could do.

In short, you went through an almost perfect system for programming and conditioning out of you your almost limitless potential and your natural programming for **achieving this potential**.

You took on board an astonishing number of rules and limits that were designed for another time and purpose – for a society that no longer exists.

But your true potential, just like the potential of the 1%, hasn't changed. The truth is that you have barely scratched the surface of what you are capable of.

THE MIND TRAP OF FALSE LIMITS

The only thing that's stopping you from getting what you want is the story you keep telling yourself.

– TONY ROBBINS

There's a great picture on Instagram of a big powerful horse that's tied up to a small plastic chair in a field. The horse has been programmed over many years that when it's tied up, it's stuck – helpless. So now all that's necessary to keep this magnificent, powerful animal completely stuck still, is a small plastic chair.

The reality is that the horse could walk away any time it liked. It's almost certainly powerful enough to break the rope and chair that's "trapping" it. But it doesn't, because it believes *the illusion of being trapped*.

This is the truth for you. Your power hasn't gone away. You always could and always will have the power and capacity to create the life you want to live and become the person you want to be. Just like the horse, all you need to do is unlearn those false limitations, the bad programming and illusions that hold you back.

So, take a few moments and consider: What limitations you have allowed into your mind that you can now let go?

What false limits, what "can'ts," what "shoulds," what lack of possibility have you unconsciously signed up to?

What your life looks like today is a direct result of the stories you tell yourself about yourself:

- About the limitations and possibilities that exist for you
- About the kind of person you are
- What kind of money someone like you makes
- How successful someone like you can be
- The kind of house someone like you lives in
- The kind of car someone like you drives
- The kind of partner and relationship someone like you deserves
- The kindness, decency, and respect someone like you deserves to get treated with
- The things that are within your reach or outside of your reach
- *About whether someone like you gets to live the life they want to live and become the person they want to be*

But here's what matters.

┌─────────────────── SIDE NOTE ───────────────────┐

This is a deliberate pattern interrupt to get you to slow down and consider. Read this section slowly and recognize that your ego will want to instantly dismiss what I've written here. Remember: change comes from considering and applying what's written, not just reading it really quickly. The challenge is to get the most benefit, not to get to the end of the book first. There are no points for finishing first. That's the Prussian education system doing its worst!

└──┘

Perception is more important than reality.

What you "know" to be possible for you matters way, way, way more than what the world believes to be "reality." Because in truth there is no such thing.

Let me give you an example to illustrate how buying into what the world calls "reality" imposes demonstrably false limits. And always remember the purpose of the education system that taught you what "reality" to buy into and why; it only wanted good, obedient soldiers and workers. It absolutely did not want people living the life of their dreams and questioning what they were told.

Sir Roger Bannister was the first man to run a mile in under four minutes. Up until he did it in 1954, most people thought the four-minute mile was impossible to break. The greatest medical and scientific minds at the time thought the human body couldn't physically run that fast.

The accepted reality was that it was "impossible." Worse than that, it was considered dangerous to try.

That was the conventional wisdom that everyone "knew" to be true. And because it was said by the brightest and cleverest among us at the time, it was accepted by almost everyone.

Roger Bannister was not a full-time professional athlete; he was a junior doctor learning his medical skills while studying at Oxford University. He didn't have much time to train; in fact, his training was minimal.

On the day of the race, the conditions were poor with winds of up to 25 miles per hour before the event. Everyone "knew" that to beat the record the conditions would have to be perfect.

But he trained his own way, fitting it around his studies and training as a doctor.

And on May 6, 1954, Roger Bannister became the first person in history to break the four-minute mile.

But here's what's interesting.

Just 46 days later, John Landy, an Australian runner, not only broke the four-minute mile but also beat Roger Bannister's time. And then over the next few years, more and more people broke through the four-minute mile and lowered the record even further – once they realized that it *was possible*.

The limits to what was possible weren't the reality everyone "knew" them to be just a few years previously. And as soon as these limits were unlearned, the previously impossible time was broken more frequently.

At the time of writing this book, the record is three minutes and 43 seconds, which is a full 17 seconds lower than Roger Bannister's time. A four-minute mile has gone from being impossible to being an average time **to being a slow time!**

There is *absolutely no difference* between the false limits the world knew existed for running a mile and those you "know" exist for you.

All of them are illusions, perceptions, and assumptions. They are not facts.

Those limits are all learned. So, they can be unlearned.

THE POWER OF THE STORIES WE TELL OURSELVES

Most people tell themselves the story that they are not "good enough" and they broadcast that story to themselves all day, every day. And so, it becomes their experience, the reality they create unconsciously, because it sets the frame for how they see the world. It defines the possibilities and opportunities that exist for them.

So, their amazing brains, the powerful supercomputer between their ears supports that perception by finding all kinds of "facts" that show it to be "true," because that's the instruction most people give their minds.

But just like the four-minute mile, not being good enough isn't a scientific fact. It's just a bullshit, sabotaging story they've told themselves.

The 1% who do achieve their goals, who do create the life they want, who do become the person they want to be, tell themselves different stories.

As you read through this, I want you to realize that there is nothing more fundamentally true about these stories that the 1% tell themselves than the bullshit limiting stories most people tell themselves.

<u>What matters is that the 1% tell themselves stories that help them, not stories that harm them.</u>

And the amazing supercomputer between their ears finds just as many "facts" to support the good story for them as it does the bad story for everyone else.

The stories the 1% tell themselves include:

- I know I'll get the life I want.
- I am naturally successful; success is inevitable for me.
- I know I deserve the best treatment in life – in love, money, respect, kindness, and sex.
- No door is closed to me.
- It would be weird for people not to treat me with kindness and respect and help me create the life I want. And if they didn't treat me well, I wouldn't want them in my life anyway.
- To get what I desire, I simply need to come up with a plan and get on with it.
- Sure, there will be challenges but that's just life (the universe, God – use whatever label works for you) helping me on my way. The challenges are there to help me, to make me stronger, not to block my path.
- There is no possibility of me not living the life that I want.

And because these are the stories they broadcast to themselves all day, every day, guess what happens?

The facts are the same, the ONLY difference is perception.

Do you now see why perception is more important than reality? Do you now see why limitations are only illusions and assumptions?

Do you now see why there is absolutely nothing more important than being able to control the thoughts in your mind, so that you can create a perception that helps you instead of one that harms you?

It's time to let go of your self-limiting stories; you no longer need to feed yourself these lies.

FUCK "SHOULD"

Until you make the unconscious conscious, it will direct your life and you will call it fate.

– CARL JUNG

How much are you living your life as the person you "should" be instead of as the person you truly are?

How much of what you do, what you feel, and what you want really comes from within you instead of in response to what society says you should feel or want?

Do the choices you've made so far align with your dreams, desires, and plans for your life? Are you living the life you chose, the life you dreamed of, on your terms? Or have you unconsciously fallen into the trap of going along with the herd, of unconsciously following the well-trodden path?

As we grow up, we develop a set of rules that define how we live and who we become. Over time these rules become internalized; they become part of who we are and the way we think. This is our "belief matrix," the set of rules and decisions that govern our whole lives; they define what we think is right and what we think works. These beliefs become *the default setting* for how we operate through life.

And because we internalize those rules, we stop consciously thinking about them; we stop considering and reviewing them. Eventually, we stop being aware that they exist.

We stop being aware that they are rules that we've given ourselves. And so most people live on autopilot, not considering if those rules are right for them or if they work against them. They become "just what you do."

The problem is that most of the rules aren't rules you've thought about, considered, or carefully chosen. They're just a default setting that you were given by your parents, siblings, teachers, friends, and society – by a whole group of people who are equally unconscious of those rules.

They form part of the group identity, part of the culture of your society, family, and group of friends. It's these rules and norms that bind you together.

And this gives rise to a very big problem.

If you decide to go against the "way things are done," you are no longer simply choosing your own path; you're not simply rejecting the rules themselves. <u>You are seen as rejecting the people, the society, that identifies with them</u>.

This is because the people around you have tied those beliefs and rules into their identity, into their sense of who they are. So, when you reject those rules, when you make your own choice, you are seen as not just rejecting the rules, but rejecting the identity of those around you.

And because you love those around you, that becomes a hard and painful thing to do. You don't wish to cause those you love pain; you don't want to feel like you are losing that connection, that common bond and identity with those you most cherish.

You are told you should follow the rules because that's the way it's always been done; you should get that job, go to college, marry "that type" of person, dress "that way," and a million other similar rules. You're told that is what you "should" be, do, and have because that's what your family, friends, teachers, and society say is "normal."

And 99% of people do exactly that.

Over time, because of societal pressure, added to by the Prussian system of education which rewards blind obedience and punishes independent thought, you stopped questioning these rules, these "shoulds."

You stopped considering whether the rules served you or worked against you, or even if they made any sense at all. They just faded to become background noise.

Up until the age of about five, children relentlessly question everything. They ask "Why?" constantly. They haven't yet taken on all the programming of the way things "should be." They shine a very bright light on all the rules in society that don't make sense. And young children naturally reject and fight against those rules.

They, just like you when you were a child, naturally focus on what makes them happy, what they want, and what works for them. They have no sense of "should."

<u>Slow down and ask yourself whether you were happier and more successful when you were a young child or now? Consider whether we should be relearning our natural confidence and successful thinking from them or whether we should be teaching them more "shoulds." Take some time to think about that</u>.

This is all part of the process of how you unlearned confidence and success, how your natural system for achieving any goal was programmed and socialized into dormancy (but importantly never lost).

Because of all this, you slowly lost touch with the real you. Because of this, you became a prisoner to thinking <u>that is designed</u> to keep you stuck, designed to stop you progressing, and designed to punish you for breaking free from this prison.

You lost touch with your dreams, and instead took on the aspirations that society says you should have. You stopped defining success on your own terms and started seeking what your society calls success, irrespective of whether that made you happy or not.

DEFINING SUCCESS ON YOUR TERMS

What does success look like to you? Slow down and attempt to not answer straightaway. Instead consider your answer.

Take a little time and think about what your life would ideally look like; what you would do with your time if you had all the money you would ever need; what your life would look like if you were free from all the traps and rules and conditioning of the "shoulds."

Below are some things to think about. Remember, there are no right or wrong answers here - there is just what would genuinely make you happy, feel good and lead you to *live your life on your terms*.

Sometimes what society says and what you want may align. And that's completely OK. The point is to consider and **become conscious** of choices most people make unconsciously - *__to re-examine the default answer and see if it's still the right answer for you.__*

As you go through these questions, don't judge yourself for taking the non-standard choice. Some of them are likely to go against the grain.

For now, be conscious of your ego when it says "there's no way I could do that." Give yourself complete freedom (maybe for the first time in years) to fully explore what you really want. This is just you exploring, free of judgement and others' expectations. So, relax. Enjoy this process. There is no rush to answer straightaway, so take as much time as you want.

- Would you like the security of a paycheck or the freedom of working for yourself? Or would you prefer to stay at home and not work? Or would you prefer to have the security of a paycheck part of the time and the freedom to work on your own business part of the time? Don't answer straightaway; just consider.
- Would you like to go to college/university or go to work (for yourself or others) as soon as possible?
- Would/does having a proper job make you happy or just feel safe?
- Do you want to get married? Or just find your perfect partner and

stay unmarried? Or would you prefer the freedom to date people in ways that suit you? Would you prefer to have multiple relationships with different people at the same time?

- Do you want children? Are you sure?
- Would you like to stay at home and look after the children or would you prefer to find a partner who would? (That's a question for both men and women to be clear!)
- Do you want a monogamous relationship or would you like to be able to have sex with whomever you want? Remember, there's no judgement so go for the answer you want.
- What sexual experiences would you like to have that you stopped looking for?
- What clothes would you like to wear or not wear?
- Would you like to live near your current friends and family or away from them? Would you like to live in one place or multiple places?
- If you could choose, would you stop working right now and go and live somewhere where you could afford not to work anymore?
- Do you like going out to parties or do you prefer to stay in and watch TV?
- Do you like all the friends you currently have?
- Do you enjoy spending time with your family?

The point of these questions is for you to become aware of how many choices you have made by default, without thought, and to start to think about whether the choices you have made make you happy or ensure your unhappiness.

I first started thinking about this when I was reading an article about Elon Musk.

In most people's eyes Elon Musk is a hero: hugely successful, with a brilliant mind. And there is absolutely no doubt that he has achieved staggering, incredible things. He is a clearly remarkable and amazing man. If anyone has "made it", he has.

But that isn't the same as having a successful life.

In an interview I saw, Elon Musk broke down crying, saying he hadn't had a week's vacation since 2001. He went on to say how he had missed much of his kids growing up and still works an average of 18 hours a day, seven days a week.

Maybe that is success to him but it isn't to me.

This is a guy worth c.$200bn who has more money than he could ever reasonably need and yet he misses his kids growing up and works 18 hours a day to the point where he nearly breaks down. I want to be clear that I am in no way judging him or his choices as that has no value to anyone.

I do want to highlight the fact that someone that the world sees as a tremendous success, leads a life that he is clearly unhappy with in important ways, despite his vast wealth and obvious success.

My point is that even with vast wealth, people still make choices based on "shoulds" rather than based on what they want. So, don't let your ego kid you that you will make different choices when you get "there."

So, consider if you want to, shifting your thinking from what you "should" do to what you want to do and what works for you.

Imagine evaluating every rule, every decision for its **benefits to you** rather than because of the perceived **obligations on you**.

But the starting point is that you have to know what **you really want** instead of what you think **you should want**. And 99% of people can't make that distinction.

So my question to you now is, do you know what you want?

Because those desires are where your true happiness lies. And once you know what they are, you can finally start working on a life that makes sense.

AND FUCK 'BEING REALISTIC'

We have been taught the lie that negative equals realistic
and positive equals unrealistic.

– SUSAN JEFFERS

I want to pick apart one of the most damaging, toxic, awful, and truly wicked pieces of bad teaching that I see almost everywhere. This way of thinking is classic accepted wisdom that is anything but wise.

This is the myth of being "realistic."

Let me start off by saying again - Fuck being realistic.

Really, tell anyone who says you need to be realistic to FUCK RIGHT OFF.

Have you fallen for this trap, for the idea that it's good and sensible to have "realistic" plans? If so, have you considered why? And more importantly, have you thought about whose definition of realistic you are using?

What most of the world considers to be realistic is really just a disguised way of saying "play small" - to give up on your dreams, to not fulfill your potential, to be, do, and have less than you otherwise could.

When people say "be realistic" what they mean is don't have big dreams, don't go after what you really want. You might fail: and you might be disappointed. Settle for something small and easy.

Just ignore for now (i.e., the rest of your life) that you've just decided to throw your dreams in the bin. **Ignore the fact that in that decision to be realistic you've just made it certain, in the only way you ever can make it certain, that you will never create the life you want to live and become the person you want to be – because you decided not to go for it.**

Do you see how toxic this is?

Without any evidence at all, you're tricked by this awful, terrible teaching of "being realistic" into limiting your success and dreams <u>before you've even got started</u>. You've unconsciously made the decision to live your life to a tiny fraction of your and its potential by falling for this lie.

Slow down for a few moments right now. Watch how your ego is likely saying all kinds of things, like:

- Being realistic is about focusing on what's possible, not fairy tales.
- It's a waste of time trying to go for something "unrealistic."
- What if going for your dreams doesn't work out, then you've wasted all of that time?
- Unless I'm realistic, I won't get anywhere at all.

And no doubt many more things just like this.

Your ego tries to fool you into thinking that you're not really capable of achieving your dreams, that they are just childhood fantasies that you need to let go of now that you're an adult, and that it will only cause you pain and disappointment to hold onto them. So stop kidding yourself and grow up and get on with living in the "real world."

Then each time something doesn't work, you think you haven't been *realistic enough,* so you scale back your dreams even further. You stop dreaming about your dream home and start thinking of that "reasonable" house that you might be able to afford. You stop looking for your perfect partner and settle for the next person you meet, because they're there and so you'd better accept that. After all, the perfect partner is just a childhood fantasy. This isn't some Disney film; this is "real life."

<u>You keep going this way, playing smaller and smaller, giving up on your dreams more and more until there's nothing left at all; until you forget that you even had dreams; until the point where you "know" that even the smallest dreams are likely to end in disappointment</u>.

Let me be clear, ***being realistic sucks***. Big time.

And it is a lie. A big, fat, toxic lie.

I know that my potential is essentially unlimited. My definition of realistic is massive, extraordinary. I refuse to put any limits on what I can achieve or how amazing my life can be. I know that whatever I dream of, I am capable of achieving.

Moreover, I know that my mind can't dream of something I am unable to achieve. The question is not whether I can but whether I desire the dream enough to do what's necessary to bring it into everyone's reality.

Stop and think about that because it is a very different way of thinking and your ego will want you to rush past this.

I'll say it again for you so it's very clear: *I know that whatever I dream of I am capable of achieving. Moreover, I know that my mind can't dream of something I am unable to achieve. The question is not whether I can, but whether I desire the dream enough to do what's necessary to bring it into everyone's reality.*

Every part of that is as true for you as it is for me.

Do you see the difference in the thinking? That shift means I'm inspired every day, open to amazing possibilities, seeing the opportunities that exist in abundance around me because I haven't shut my mind off to them by deciding that they're not realistic.

I haven't shut the door on amazing things, incredible abundance, wonderful experiences and people and a life aligned to my dreams just because someone who has given up on their dreams thinks I'm being unrealistic. No way.

So right now, I expect your ego is kicking off in a big way, saying that it's all very well someone like me saying this, but you don't have time for woo-woo fantasies, that you "have to" live in the real world, that those dreams might happen for other people but not for you, and so on and so on.

So let me explain why this lie of being realistic is completely flawed.

To be clear, the notion that expecting a negative outcome is realistic is complete and utter bullshit.

It is an inaccurate, toxic, damaging thought that keeps you playing small but is nonetheless one that most of the world has accepted as a fact.

Great things, overflowing abundance, in your work, in your love life, with your health are all every bit as realistic as the negative stuff.

In fact, it's your natural state.

If you (by which I mean your ego) instinctively reacted against that last sentence, then be grateful that you've just realized that you've fallen for the lie that bad stuff is realistic and you've found something that's blocking you from getting your dreams.

Here's how this works.

Your mind is a perceptual machine. This is why perception is more important than "reality". What that means is that what you perceive to be true, becomes true.

So if your dominant thoughts about you and your life are that you're lucky, that great things happen to you and that you live in a grateful, happy, abundant, and inspired state then your life will reflect that.

Good things, great things, and miracles will happen to you. All the time.

Whereas if you "know" that only the bad stuff in life is realistic, then your subconscious mind will find amazing and inventive ways of making that your reality.

Whether you realize it or not, whether you believe it or not, those thoughts and feelings are the way you communicate "what you want" to your subconscious mind.

If you buy into the "negative equals realistic" lie, you've literally told your subconscious mind to create lots of negative realism in your life. You probably have way more of this stuff in your life right now than you'd like.

Do you see how important this is now?

This isn't some woo-woo nonsense. This is how the supercomputer between your ears actually works. Just because nearly the whole world doesn't understand this or dismisses it doesn't make it any less true.

One of my favorite quotes is, "The truth is the truth even if no one believes it. A lie is a lie even if everyone believes it."

You can choose to continue to believe the lie, as almost the entire world does. And you'll get the same results as nearly everyone else.

Or you can choose to believe the truth, even though it goes completely against the grain, that your dreams are not only possible but entirely realistic and you've just been using your mind incorrectly.

One thought helps you, the other one harms you.

I'll be going through how to use your mind to get exactly what you want later in the book. Don't skip ahead for that part: it will come in the right time and the right way.

I've designed this book very carefully to give you exactly what you need in the right order. So just relax and enjoy the part that you're learning right now: this is where your confidence and success get created.

DO YOU FEEL WORTHY OF SUCCESS?

We will act consistently with our view of who we truly are, whether that view is accurate or not.

– TONY ROBBINS

What kind of life do you feel you deserve?

What kind of success, relationships, money, respect, health, friendships, love do you feel you are worthy of?

Do you know you <u>deserve</u> the very best of what life has to offer or do you just want it?

Do you, like many people, feel that you do not really deserve the best? I mean, it would be nice but it's just not the kind of thing that happens for someone like me.

This feeling isn't necessarily a specific thought like "I don't deserve this" or "I don't deserve to feel good about myself." But rather, it's far more often a question: "What makes me think I deserve good things, deserve to feel good about myself? **What makes me think I'm worth the effort?**"

This is one of the single biggest stumbling blocks to people becoming who they want to be and living the life they want to live. It places a complete block on your progress and is the core underlying basis for **nearly all self-sabotage**.

All your attempts to progress, to grow, to become more, to create the life you want will be sabotaged and undermined by any sense you have that you don't deserve the good outcome.

You will act (by which I mean self-sabotage) consistently with your view that you do not deserve the best.

This is an insidious and incredibly toxic mind trap that huge numbers of people fall for and spend their entire lives trapped by. It's why so many people who make sincere and genuine efforts to improve their lives trip themselves up, sabotage their own success, and get in their own way.

It's why so many people can find success in fleeting ways and then seem to only and inevitably backslide. They "know" they don't deserve the success they desire, they expect, and are often just waiting for whatever success they do create to be taken away or to be balanced out by something bad in some other area of their life.

The process can be so insidious and subtle that most people don't realize that it's happening.

Maybe you don't complete what you started, or start off well and then your focus, effort, and attention somehow just fall away. You get distracted or somehow you get too busy at work, with friends, a phone call, or something on TV and your progress slows and eventually halts. Your ego tells you that you "had" to do these other things.

People sabotage their own success in relationships, in business, with friends, and in their own development.

Fear of success comes from feeling undeserving of success.

If you don't feel deserving, you will find a way of not allowing yourself to have it, whatever it may be. Your concept of yourself as undeserving compels you to sabotage, retreat from, and resist the very experiences, changes, and success you long for.

And it becomes a horrible vicious cycle. Each new failure (no matter that it resulted from self-sabotage) is yet more false evidence for your ego to use the next time you try to create your dreams.

Here's how this works.

Each of us has a mental self-portrait that defines who we are and the way we think and feel about ourselves. That portrait is the result of your past experiences, successes, failures, feelings, and behaviors. It's the foundation upon which our view of ourselves and our place in the world is constructed.

That mental self-portrait sets the frame for what we expect to happen in our lives and consciously or unconsciously we act in accordance with it.

Do you ever wonder why some people who are incredibly talented, gifted, kind, honest, caring and decent don't get what they desire in life while others who are far less talented, far less gifted, just seem to have things fall into place for them?

The difference is what they expect and what they know they deserve.

Those expectations create their reality just as your expectations create yours.

Most people have distorted mental self-portraits because through bad teaching and programming they have been taught to focus on and to expect the negative, to expect things not to work out, to go wrong, to not last. They've been taught that they can't, that they are not worthy, that they don't deserve, that they're not skilled enough and so on.

And so, they unconsciously feel that they are not worthy of success. And as a result, their subconscious mind **which is your perfect servant**, creates exactly that for you.

Remember that your subconscious mind acts in accordance with the feelings you feed it not the words.

So if you feed it with feeling of a lack of worthiness and deserving, it will go and find and create ample experiences in your life where things happen to reinforce that view.

Slow down and consider for a moment, is your lack of deservingness a fact, an obvious and inherent truth? When you objectively consider it, are you obviously and clearly less worthy, less deserving than others around you?

When you look at a young child starting off in the world, with all their beautiful innocence and joy, do you decide there and then that they don't deserve the great, the wonderful, the joyous things in life? Do you decide that they are unworthy?

It seems completely ridiculous to say it or even consider it. It feels like a self-evident truth that the beautiful child deserves a wonderful life because...just because.

And yet you were once that young child.

And I promise you that many adults, weary with their own feelings of unworthiness, looked at you then (and look at you now) and think exactly those thoughts.

Young children instinctively and naturally assume they deserve whatever they want. They haven't yet been taught not to. When they grab a toy that isn't theirs, food that they want, when they go up to strangers and smile at them, do you think they shouldn't because they don't deserve those things?

Do you think they don't deserve all the love, wonder, and attention that they get? Do you see any lack of self-worth, any sense at all in a young child that they don't deserve what they want?

There is no truth, despite what your ego and most of the world would tell you, in any sense that you don't deserve, in any lack of worthiness. The belief that you are not worthy or that you don't deserve "it," whatever it may be, is complete and total bullshit.

As T Harv Eker says, it's a "I don't have to try" pill.

If I don't do well, it's OK because I'm not worthy anyway. If you want to block success, if you want to block the pure greatness, joy and gifts within you, all you have to do is tell yourself the bullshit lie that that you're "unworthy" and it's done. It gives you a nice excuse for your life, but it doesn't in anyway help you become who you want to be and create the life you want to live. Don't kid yourself differently.

You unlearned the natural sense of self-worth and deservingness that you had as a child. So it can just as easily be relearned. It's only a matter of shining the light on the false, inaccurate belief of unworthiness.

You don't need to try to change your beliefs, you only need to realize the truth.

THINGS TO CONSIDER

- Can you see that your true potential (like everyone else's) is way, way, way more than most people can conceive?

- Consider that the only thing blocking you from accessing and unleashing that incredible potential is a false sense of limitation.

- Consider how perception is more important than reality. Can you see this as the truth?

- Can you see how controlling your thoughts controls your perception of yourself and the wider world – and so controls your success?

- Consider how the traditional education system set you up to fail, not succeed. Consider how much you have achieved despite being taught a near-perfect system for failure.

- Consider what the real meaning of "being realistic" is for most of the world. Consider whether this definition of realistic has helped you or harmed you. And consider whether you want to change your definition of realistic to expecting the best instead of playing small.

- Consider how a false and distorted perception of who you are, driven by your ego and supported by bad teaching, has held you back. Can you see how this false self-perception is based on lies?

CHAPTER 5

LETTING GO OF DESTRUCTIVE EMOTIONAL BAGGAGE

Life is a journey and you can't carry everything with you. Only take the usable baggage.

HA JIN

At the start of this book, I told you that becoming confident, becoming who you want to be, and creating the life you want to live, isn't about learning anything.

That it is instead about unlearning and letting go of the destructive teaching and the resulting emotional baggage that 99% of the people in the world carry with them. And that then your natural, unstoppable mindset is free to run your life again.

That "baggage" is all the negative, harmful thoughts and feelings from your past – all the guilt, all the shame, all the pain, regret, and heartache.

So many go through life, through each experience they face, picking up more and more baggage to carry with them. More pain, more guilt, and more regret.

Until eventually they are so buried by that baggage, they can't even see who they are any more.

Their journey is hard and exhausting; each step forward is a massive effort because they are so weighed down by all the painful, emotional baggage they are carrying with them.

Over time they create a bond with this pain, they identify with it until it becomes part of who they are. They identify as people who have "suffered" and pain and suffering are what they come to expect. They come to think that holding onto all of that pain and suffering makes them smarter and wiser.

And for their ego, that pain becomes a fortress.

A fortress of pain and bad feelings that keep you safe, protecting you from anyone ever hurting you again. **But this ignores the obvious fact that you are hurting yourself over and over again by holding onto the pain and regret**; that you are trapping yourself in that pain, in your past, and never truly moving forwards into the life you want and deserve.

The trick to life, as Andy taught me, is to progress through life with just baggage enough: to carry with you the lessons and the benefits from all your experiences.

To progress only with the ___resources___ that help you be who you want to be, not with the ___baggage___ that stops you from ever living the life you want.

This isn't what most people do. In fact, most people do ***exactly the opposite of this***. They hold on tightly to the pain, the regret, the sense of failure and loss, and never even look for - let alone find - the benefits of all the experiences they have had.

WHY FEEL BAD?

I want to introduce you to one of the most powerful mindsets that the 1% use.

This goes seriously against the grain of how almost the entire world thinks and even more importantly how 99% of people think you should think.

Recognize, for a moment, that the way the 99% think doesn't help you create the life of your dreams and in fact blocks you completely from living life on your terms.

But here's the problem.

What I'm about to tell you is simple. Like, really simple. And that should be a good thing. <u>But it actually ends up working against you, unless you slow down enough to properly consider what is being said.</u>

Your ego will try to say "Well that's obvious" or "I know that already" conveniently ignoring the fact that you "knowing" this doesn't mean you have applied it in your life in any way. And so, it's actually been completely useless to you.

I'm going to ask you one simple question.

Why feel bad?

Don't look for what your mind says, look for your feelings when you read this question. Feel your answer.

What is the purpose, value, or benefit of you feeling bad in any way?

Who does this help? Whose life is improved? Whose feelings are soothed? What does this change for the better?

What I'd like you to do now is put this book down for a few minutes and just consider this. As always, it's your choice whether you do this or not, but as I've said several times, **the way you change and actually get the most benefit from this book comes from considering what's written, not from reading through the book as quickly as possible.**

There are no prizes for finishing the book first. But there is a prize for getting the most benefit, and that prize is the life you want and becoming who you want to be.

So, give yourself a few minutes and just think through all the things you feel or have felt bad about and consider what good resulted from you feeling bad? Don't try to come up with the "right" answer or the answer you think you should have, but look to understand if there were any benefits there at all.

⌛

So, did you do the exercise or did you just read on?

If you did the exercise, you most likely struggled to find a true, real, tangible benefit. Most people come up with answers such as "It shows that I care / am a good person / not a sociopath / have feelings" or "Feeling bad stops me from making the same mistake again."

But consider, why does feeling bad help this? Why is it necessary to feel bad to care? Is it really true that you need to feel guilty, or full of pain and regret to be a good person? Even if you did something bad or hurt someone, do your feelings of guilt heal that in any way? Does your guilt change what happened?

The notion that you should feel bad for your mistakes, the things you got wrong, or the pain you caused, is wrong even if it's what 99% of people believe and wider society tells you is true. <u>We have been fed the lie that you cannot be considered a kind, decent, caring person if you don't feel guilt, pain, anguish, regret, and shame.</u>

And as a result, so many people live nearly their entire lives carrying these bad feelings with them which wreaks terrible damage on their lives and their ability to create the life they want.

But imagine for a second if you dropped all of those bad feelings. Imagine if, instead, you focused all of your energy, all of that emotion into simply doing what you could to make the situation better and then learning the lessons from that experience.

Imagine as well if those who suffered from whatever pain you may have caused also only looked for the benefit to them of their experience - that instead of becoming victims of the experience they simply took all of the benefit and dropped all of the pain.

Imagine if in every bad experience you ever faced, in every wrong ever done to you, you could automatically sift through the experience and take all the knowledge, all the wisdom, all the learning, all the things that would help you and then leave everything else behind, because it had no value to you.

Let me give you an example to show you what I mean.

Think of a marriage break up, where one person has an affair and it causes the break-up of that relationship. The infidelity creates enormous pain and heartache to the other person, a massive breach of trust, an end to all that they have built together, the life that they worked so hard for. Years of life together broken apart at enormous emotional and financial cost for a fleeting mistake.

Even imagine that there are young children involved, who are completely innocent and now face the pain of seeing their world turned upside down, the end of their secure family unit, the loss of their home, witnessing the arguments between their parents, the anger and hurt they see in each of their parents.

Imagine all of this pain resulted from a mistake <u>or even a deliberate choice</u>.

Now that it has happened, how does your partner, how do your children, how do you benefit in any way from you feeling bad? I get that this completely goes against everything you've been taught, against everything nearly everyone will tell you, but that doesn't make it true.

I want to be completely clear that I'm not suggesting for a second that if you've been unfaithful to your partner that you don't have a lot of work to do to remediate the situation. I'm not suggesting you should be emotionless and unfeeling at the loss of your marriage or the hurt feelings of your partner or children.

What I am saying is that the very best thing you can do in that situation is focus 100% of your energy, your time, and effort on creating the best possible outcome from that position for those you love and yourself.

And every tiny bit of energy given over to feeling bad detracts from that effort and results in a worse outcome for everyone. It means less effort available to create the best outcome and a little bit more lost and wasted on feelings of regret, grief, and remorse that serve no useful purpose.

The 1% do this naturally. They know or rather they never forgot to seek and find the benefit in every situation they face. They know that feeling bad has no value.

They know it is pointless, a waste of time and energy that will simply slow them down on their journey through life. <u>They know that the only reason to experience anything, the only thing to seek out is the lesson, the experience that will make them stronger, wiser and better equipped as they progress.</u>

They go forward with the resources from every experience and drop everything else.

They know everything else they carry is simply excess weight that not only doesn't help them but actively harms them. They know it isn't something that just passively sits at the back of their mind - it is a cancer that eats away at their dreams, desires and most importantly at their self-esteem.

You once did this too, when you were a young child, before you had been taught that you "should" feel bad when things went wrong or when you did something you "shouldn't."

Look at a young child when they make a mistake, hurts another child, or gets hurt. In the moment, they are upset. But quickly and naturally they move past those emotions, <u>return to the present moment</u> (where all living is done) and carry on as if nothing much has happened. They simply deal with the immediate situation in front of them.

A few minutes after they have dealt with the immediate upset, they are cracking on with their lives, enjoying the moment, having adventures. They aren't carrying hurt, pain, or anger with them.

The 1% never forgot how to do this, how to live this way, the way you were designed to live naturally.

You may have unlearned this and forgotten it, but you can't lose this ability. It is your default programming. Right now, it is simply dormant, lying there within your DNA waiting to be re-activated.

Next, I want to go through some of the common negative baggage that most people carry with them and show you how to let it all go.

WHY YOU NEVER NEED TO FEEL GUILTY AGAIN

Guilt does not change the past. Guilt doesn't make the future better. Guilt does not help others or ourselves. Guilt does not fix problems. Guilt blinds us from the ability to change, grow and improve. It's time to let go of guilt.

– JESSICA ORTNER

How much of your time do you spend feeling guilty about things you have done in the past?

How do you feel about the fact that you may still feel guilty about things that you said or did, days, weeks, months, or even years ago? How much of your life have you given over to guilt, to things that you cannot change?

Guilt is a deeply toxic thought pattern that causes untold misery. It isn't natural and isn't something that has ANY place in your life.

The idea that you should feel guilty is so normalized that it's not something anyone really questions.

But always be aware of herd mentality thinking and whether this thinking is just accepted wisdom (which is rarely wise and rarely helpful) or just something people have decided is so obviously true that they've switched off their minds.

At its core, guilt is a mind trap that is truly awful, not just for the person feeling guilty but equally for those they love and the wider world. It is a way of thinking that inevitably and only *lessens* the amount of good, the amount of happiness, and the amount of joy in the world.

It's a trap that virtually guarantees that anyone caught in it, cannot and will not fulfil their incredible potential. This means that all of their gifts, all of their experience, all of the lessons they have learned from the experience that the world says they should feel guilty about – all of this goes to waste.

The cancer at the heart of guilt is the notion that you cannot be a good person unless you feel bad for the things that you have done; that if you don't feel guilty, you "must" be uncaring, unfeeling, and even some kind of sociopath.

Here's why this is so damaging and why people find it hard to break out of this mind trap.

You know you are a good person and because you "know" that, good people feel guilty when you do something "bad" or "wrong" – that means that you "must" feel some kind of guilt for all of the mistakes, miscalculations, moments of weakness, mis-steps, and flashes of anger you've ever had.

If they don't feel guilty then by definition you are a bad person, unkind or nasty. The more guilt you feel, the longer you feel it, the less you ever truly forgive yourself, the more of a good person you are.

So, the process of becoming and remaining a good person requires you beat yourself up as much as possible, to cause yourself as much pain as possible.

This is the insane thought that the only path to being and demonstrating that you are a good person is through feeling bad.

Most people wonder why they can't let the past go – well this is why. Because to let it go would at a subconscious level mean admitting you were secretly a bad person all along!

And so, you stay trapped in this guilt from the moment you are socialized into believing this bullshit until the day you either set yourself free (hint: today is a good day to do that) or when you die.

If this was someone else doing this to you, it would be called a toxic, emotionally abusive relationship. Well, it is toxic and abusive, it's just that you are doing it to yourself.

Unfortunately, the damage doesn't stop there.

I repeat many times throughout this book that every person has unique and wonderful gifts, and that the purpose of life is to find your true calling, to unleash your gifts, your unique experiences, and all the lessons you have learned for the benefit of yourself, and of those you love and the world around you.

Now consider: How much harder do you think it is for you or anyone to do that when you're carrying the heavy baggage of years of guilt? How can you feel that you are worthy of unleashing your gifts if you're caught in ***the toxic trap of "trying" to be good by feeling bad?***

Does feeling guilty make any sense AT ALL?

HOW GUILT SCREWED ME UP

Let me give you a personal example of the damage that guilt does.

A long time ago when I was at university, I cheated on a girlfriend I had at the time. I loved her very much; we were deeply in love and for a long time I thought we would get married.

What happened was entirely my fault and I had no good reason for doing it.

As a result of what I did, she was deeply hurt and felt completely betrayed. And she had every right to feel that way. Our relationship deteriorated directly as a result and we ultimately broke up.

At the time I felt awful for what I had done. I felt terrible over the pain I had caused someone I loved, someone who had always been kind and loving towards me and who hadn't done anything to deserve that betrayal. And I felt even worse over the fact that we broke up. I knew it was my fault. It took me a long time to get over the end of that relationship. I carried the guilt of that for a long time.

Now here's where this bites.

Because I carried that guilt with me (instead of just the lessons) I ended up making a series of pretty terrible relationship choices and I stuck with them because of not wanting to repeat the guilt. That ended up causing me, my future girlfriends and those closest to me a lot of pain, grief, and general heartache.

And I spent a lot more time feeling pretty awful about myself as a result.

Feeling guilty simply created more experiences in my life to feel guilty for.

Only when I realized this awful trap and I truly let the guilt go did things start to change.

Only when I broke the vicious cycle of guilt, when I saw the truth that I was a good person, a human being who was imperfect and fallible, but with good intentions, could I start to make much better "guilt free" choices.

So take some time to really look at the guilt you're carrying. Understand the costs that your guilt is having to your life right now and the costs it will carry on having until you put this baggage down.

Decide whether you can now just take forward the lessons and the benefits instead of carrying the guilt the world says you should. Decide if you want to do anything to make amends for things you may have done in your past, but do this without expectation of recognition. Just do it because it's who you are.

Then let guilt go.

You don't need it anymore and the world needs the very best you not the you suffocating under years of guilt.

TOXIC SHAME

I want to touch briefly on toxic shame. This is the stage on from chronic guilt.

Because if you carry your guilt for long enough the cancer of guilt metastasizes into shame.

It is the shift from thinking "I did something bad" to "I am bad."

It's the thought pattern that says I not only did something wrong but that I am wrong to my core - broken, bad, defective, and unlovable.

What results is a sense that you can only experience acceptance and love if you hide that shameful part of yourself away; that if you do not disguise who you really are, you will be found out and your "true unlovability" will be revealed.

It is impossible to feel truly good about who you are or to like yourself if you feel shame about yourself. So you hide that part of yourself away and then you feel more ashamed because you know you are not being honest about who you are.

You feel that if people like you, **it's only because they don't know the truth about you**. This causes you to keep that part of you buried deeper out of fear that if the real you is discovered then you will lose that friendship or love.

And so, the vicious cycle continues.

The antidote to all of this is honesty and authenticity. By accepting and revealing all of who you are, all of your rough edges and imperfections, you set yourself free. And in doing so you allow others to do the same.

More on that later.

THE PROBLEM WITH PERFECTIONISM

Perfectionism is not the same thing as striving to be your best. Perfectionism is the belief that if we live perfect, look perfect and act perfect, we can minimize or avoid the pain of blame, judgement and shame. It's a shield. It's a twenty-ton shield that we lug around thinking it will protect us when, in fact, it's the thing preventing us from flight.

– BRENÉ BROWN

Do you hear people say proudly that they are a perfectionist? That they hold themselves to a standard of perfection in all that they think, say, or do? That being perfect is somehow the pinnacle of human achievement?

Maybe you think this too.

If so, why do you think that this is a noble aspiration? Why do you strive for perfection in anything? Could this be another thing that you have come to accept and believe without thought?

Most people are taught that they "should" aim for perfection, that somehow it makes them better and more successful if they are never satisfied until they attain perfection in something.

But what if this is wrong? Or what if it is not simply wrong, but actually toxic and self-destructive?

What if this is another piece of bad teaching that is blocking your natural confidence and success?

Perfectionism is a destructive and addictive belief system that is based on the false assumption that if you **_appear_** perfect and do everything perfectly then you can avoid judgement or minimize feelings of shame or judgement.

The tragedy is that the desire to appear perfect fatally undermines your chances of success. It takes you in precisely the *opposite* direction of where you're trying to go.

The false teaching is that by aiming for perfection you will hit greater highs, achieve more, become more. Yet all the research shows the opposite. Rather than pushing you ever higher, the research shows that it is the path to depression, anxiety, addiction, and life paralysis.

Which you may have noticed, isn't exactly perfect.

The magic ingredient for success in anything is momentum. The quicker you take action on something you've learned or want to achieve, the more likely you are to succeed. Because it's only by taking action, making mistakes and applying the lesson that you learn and grow.

But if you focus on being perfect and not making mistakes, you can't learn the lessons you need to learn and you can't move to the next stage.

Because life gives you the lessons you need through making mistakes.

Children know this instinctively and you once did too. As a child when you got a new toy or saw your friends playing a new game, did you read the instruction manual or the rules cover to cover? Or did you just go and play, make mistakes, and learn through doing? The reason children play is that's how they learn: by doing – by having fun, <u>by making mistakes</u>, and finding out what works.

The ultimate goal isn't to be perfect. It's happiness. Happiness is the only reason to ultimately do anything. And happiness comes from accepting, liking, and enjoying who you are without reference to other people's false standards and measures.

Happiness means finding and living to your true purpose. It means making your life an adventure where you explore just how far you can go. It means recognizing that you, like every human being that has ever lived, has "flaws."

Perfectionism distracts you from being the real you, which is where your happiness lies. It blocks you from being who you really are, saying what you really think, liking what you really like, and doing what you really want to do.

It stops you from being real.

Perfectionism is really just a fear of failure by another name. But the truth is that someone, somewhere will always find fault, will find some lack of "perfection" with you.

It is literally impossible to please all of the people all of the time. And often it's pretty hard to please some of the people some of the time.

When you truly understand this, when you go from intellectually knowing it to applying it and then living it as a way of life, it is incredibly liberating.

You are free to be real instead of perfect, to be authentic instead of fake. You free yourself to make the mistakes that are an essential part of the human experience, no matter how much people pretend otherwise.

Then and only then can true learning, true confidence, and true success begin.

It is your rough edges that make you human. They are your friends; they are not to be feared or hidden away.

Perfectionism is the fast track to misery. Put down the heavy piece of baggage, this need to be without flaw – it's not possible and it's not even a good aim.

WHEN YOU COMPARE YOU DESPAIR

The first step to accepting yourself is to stop comparing yourself to others

– JOE DUNCAN

Comparison isn't just the thief of joy it's the thief of everything – your joy, your confidence, your self-esteem, your success and your peace of mind. And it gives you nothing in return.

As my friends Richard Wilkins and Liz Ivory say, **when you compare you despair.**

Comparison makes you feel inferior or superior. But both of these are a waste of time and neither serve any useful purpose at all. Even when you feel superior you've still fallen for the same mind trap of comparison and soon enough someone will come along who makes you feel shit about who you are.

Most people spend (by which I mean waste) huge amounts of time comparing themselves to others; deciding if they measure up or down; deciding if what they have, who they are, what they've achieved, the life they have, the partner they're with, and so on and so on is better or worse than someone else's.

This is a truly awful way to live.

Consider what benefit there is in comparing yourself to others in any way. When you compare yourself to someone you "believe" is doing better than you, does this help you on your journey to becoming the person you want to be and living the life you want to live? Or does it simply make you feel inadequate, and slow you down?

When you compare, you are assuming that you are on the same journey as someone else. But you're not – you're on <u>your journey</u>. So, what if by trying to be better than someone else you only think you've progressed, when in fact you've simply wandered further off track.

Because their track and their journey aren't your track and your journey.

So now you've worked really hard to go in the wrong direction.

Imagine what would happen if you focused on your own journey instead of others'. Imagine if instead of recalibrating your thoughts, feelings, actions and choices to what someone else did, you simply made sure you took a step forward, big or small on your journey each day.

Imagine if what others did only served as inspiration for you, to show you what was possible for you instead of making you feel like you have in some way fallen short?

<u>Comparing yourself to others is a game you cannot win, because by definition someone else sets the rules and the goal.</u>

Confident, successful people know this instinctively. One of the defining characteristics of true confidence is that the idea of comparing yourself to others just seems...well, a little silly.

What the 1% feel or think about themselves is in no way affected by what anyone else is, what anyone else does, or what anyone has. Joining the 1% club is a simple, calm, serene knowing that you are enough, that you can, and that you are worthy and deserving of the best in life.

It isn't arrogance that you are somehow better than someone else. There's a very, very big difference between confidence and arrogance.

And that difference is consciousness.

Confident people are perfectly aware of their flaws. But they accept them completely: **they own them**. They don't fear them or need to hide them away. They love, like, and accept themselves in totality, and that is where that calm strength comes from.

Those who are arrogant and look down on others are really weak-minded people who can only feel good by trying to make themselves superior to others. Their feelings about themselves cannot be sustained without comparison to others.

Only by showing how others are flawed are they able to access their own sense of worth.

This is pure weakness, disguised (badly) as strength – weakness that requires power over others to be sustained and survive. It is too weak on its own. This is tyranny, not confidence.

Stop playing the comparison game. It is a game that cannot be won. There is no benefit to it.

As Cheryl Richardson says, "You will never feel motivated to do more by feeling less than." The only way to win is to not play the game.

THINGS TO CONSIDER

- Consider: Is there any value or benefit at all in you feeling bad in any way?

- Consider whether you are carrying any destructive emotional baggage (bad feelings) that you no longer need.

- Can you see that you can be a good person and do the most good for yourself and others by letting go of all destructive emotional baggage?

- Consider how quickly you would make progress if you only took the benefit (the resources) from every experience and left all the bad feelings behind.

- Consider if there is any benefit to you in ever feeling guilty again.

- Consider if you need to feel guilty to do whatever is right and necessary to heal any pain or harm that you may have caused. Or can you just do it by simply being conscious and aware?

- Consider how perfectionism blocks the natural process for success by causing you to fear making mistakes.

- Can you see that by comparing yourself to others, you are sending yourself on the wrong journey – someone else's journey. So that even if you win the comparison game, you've still lost.

- Consider if you ever want to compare yourself to others again.

CHAPTER 6

CURING THE CANCER OF PEOPLE PLEASING

Care about what people think and you will always be their prisoner.

LAO TZU

If there was one behavior that I would like to rid the world of, it is people pleasing: the debilitating sense that your role, your purpose should be, in any way, to "please" another. Or that in order to "be OK," you require the approval of someone else.

There is nothing as devastating to your self-esteem as people pleasing and approval seeking.

Nothing else comes even close.

It is the fast track to <u>blocking and limiting the potential for your life</u> because the agenda for your life is almost entirely set by what you think other people want, instead of independently creating your life in a way that makes sense for you.

It causes <u>you to lose touch with what you want</u>, with your authentic values and your true choices. It causes you to sacrifice the essence of your life through the fear of rejection and disapproval – sometimes from one person in particular, sometimes from those around you in general.

It causes you to <u>stop communicating honestly</u>. After all, if you say what you really want, that could get rejected. Or instead of simply, calmly, and kindly saying no to things that you don't want and don't agree with, people pleasers say yes to all manner of obligations and then find petty excuses in order to get out of them.

You know you're lying, and those around you almost certainly know you're lying too.

People pleasing makes you anxious, because you have no framework for stopping people crossing your boundaries and getting you to do things you don't want to do. It puts you at the mercy of any request from someone else because you lack the emotional infrastructure (the internal "integrity") to say no. And so everyone around you represents another potential unwanted obligation or boundary infringement.

It creates a huge web of resentments because the people pleaser feels like they sacrifice everything for others and get little in return. And those around them dislike the lies and hidden obligations that come with every interaction – that sense that they somehow need to say "Well done" or gush with approval for every act of kindness from the people pleaser.

It becomes a vicious cycle of seeking affirmation, approval, and positive feedback from those around you, by catering to their needs and obliging to their wishes. And as you increasingly lose sense of who you really are without that approval you crave it even more.

Soon enough people pleasers and approval seekers lose all sense of themselves. They don't know who they are without that approval and validation. They certainly don't have any internal, independent sense of validation and approval. They need a constant *external* supply.

Do you see how and why this is such a cancer in most people's lives?

Can you see how it is impossible to even *be you* until you let this go?

MY STORY WITH PEOPLE PLEASING

I have had an interesting and slightly complex relationship with people pleasing. I am not a natural people pleaser but there have certainly been times where I have fallen into this trap.

And I have been the target of people pleasers and experienced just how grating it can be.

That perspective has given me a wonderful insight into why this is the worst behavior possible for your confidence and success.

Towards the end of my marriage I unquestionably became a people pleaser and approval seeker with my ex-wife. I bent over backwards, forwards, sideways, and every other way, in order to keep her happy and to try to hold our relationship (and so our family) together.

My decision-making process for almost everything became focused on whether it would upset her, make her happy, help or harm what little was left of our relationship. I was treading on eggshells, anxious and on edge the entire time.

And all it (rightly) did was accelerate the end of our relationship. I wasn't respecting myself and I wasn't being authentic. In fact, I was being pretty pathetic. There could never be any respect or attraction, because I was not acting in respectful or attractive ways.

Equally, I have had times when I have had a very successful personal life and relationships. Those relationships were successful because I was authentic; I was self-respecting, I was giving in the relationship not to please but simply because it was who I was.

I had no agenda or expectation of anything in return.

Nothing about the person I was or the way I was acting had <u>anything</u> to do with getting the approval of the person I was with. It had everything to do with me living authentically and in alignment with my values. I communicated honestly what I thought and felt. I knew what I wanted and what made me happy and I encouraged equally clear communication in return – *because I didn't need their approval or fear their disapproval*.

And so, we were both free to be who we really were and those relationships were highly successful.

I have also been in (short-lived) relationships with people pleasers and it caused me to understand how unpleasant and unenjoyable an experience it is.

I once went out with someone who seemed great at first. She seemed kind, caring, affectionate, and beautiful. But I saw how the "kind" things she did were really just set-ups to get what she wanted in return.

Kind things were done unexpectedly (which was great) but were usually followed by some kind of indirect request for something else. It was pretty transparent why the kind thing had been done. The bigger the act of "kindness," the bigger the request or expectation there was in return. After all, she had done "all of these amazing things for me."

Except she hadn't done it **for me** at all. She had done it to get something **from me**.

Whether that was a progression in the relationship I wasn't ready for, a night out "in return," or some extra level of communication to tell her she was "amazing or wonderful," each act of kindness always came with a hidden price tag.

Now don't get me wrong: it's great to do wonderful things for the people you like and love. But these are only kindnesses if you do them without expectation or agenda.

It very quickly got to the stage where each act of trying to please me (instead of just being an amazing partner for its own sake) built resentments.

I felt manipulated and came to resist and resent the future kind acts and view all others with some degree of suspicion. She came to resent me for not "paying her back" for all the kind things she had done.

And the relationship quickly died.

Can you see how destructive this behavior is? How it breaches trust and stacks resentments?

WHY APPROVAL SEEKING AND PEOPLE PLEASING IS SO HARD TO GIVE UP

When it is pointed out to them, most people can see fairly quickly and easily just how damaging and destructive approval seeking is to their lives and their sense of well-being. But despite **intellectually understanding** this, they struggle to <u>apply it</u> and so to fully give up the need to please others.

What begins as a learned behavior becomes an ingrained habit. And the habit crystallizes into a default setting, something done on autopilot.

But approval seeking is still a learned behavior, <u>not a natural behavior</u>. Your natural successful way of thinking hasn't disappeared. Your operating system has just been given a bad bit of software to run.

Because you learned it, you can **unlearn it** and remove this bad programming from your mind. But doing so requires two things: for you to be conscious of when you try to please others and to understand the subconscious beliefs and thinking patterns that cause you to do this in the first place.

By shining a light on the false assumptions, the inaccurate, toxic beliefs that underpin this behavior, you remove the foundations that keep it in place. And once you remove the foundations, then you <u>naturally and without effort</u> revert to your natural success and confidence mindset.

THE TOXIC MYTHS OF PEOPLE PLEASING

One of the biggest blocks to people giving up approval seeking is that they think that <u>pleasing others makes them a good person</u>. And that if they stop, they will somehow become a bad person.

They think that pleasing others <u>is the same as being kind to others</u> – it is not.

They think that pleasing others is <u>bringing good into the world</u> – it is not.

And they think that pleasing others and getting their approval will somehow help them – but it helps you in <u>none of the ways that matter</u> and works against you in *all of the ways that do*.

Here's the problem.

Your ego takes something that appears good and noble (doing good by others, trying to make others happy) and turns it into a weapon, by making your sense of your own value dependent on how much you please other people.

So "doing good" quickly transmutes into subservience.

That means you weren't actually being as kind and decent as most people think. You were, in truth, ***engaging in a trade*** that the other person didn't know that they were part of. ***You were seeking their validation as a payment for your "good" deeds.***

People pleasing is an approach to life that says <u>you're not enough on your own</u> – that your worth only exists as a function of the validation and feedback you get from others.

If others say you're OK then all is right with the world. If others say that you're wrong, no matter how baseless and invalid the reasons, then your sense of self gets crushed, because it doesn't have solid foundations.

As a people pleaser, everything that defines your life, its meaning, and its success becomes filtered through the lens of what will make someone else happy. You bend yourself out of shape, mentally, physically, and emotionally in order to fit in – ***which really means to blend in, to disappear into the background.***

The idea that you need to be something you're not, think things you don't, say things you don't mean and literally change the person you are in order to comply with someone else's idea of what you should be, is insane.

It doesn't get any less insane just because so many people live this way.

That's because for many *people pleasing is an addiction*.

It becomes addictive because, over time, pleasing others (and so being a "good" person) becomes part of your identity. It becomes who you are and what you do. And you've been told that it makes you a kind, decent person; it means you're respecting the values that your parents gave you. So, to not do it means you'd not be a good person and you'd be disrespecting your parents.

Can you see how this works?

The more successful you are at people pleasing, the more you give up your own identity. It slowly erodes away the rest of your identity, the rest of your individuality, until you forget who you really are.

If you no longer independently have your own thoughts, your own ideas, your own choices – if they only exist for you as an extension of what pleases others – then without that approval, you literally disappear. Soon enough you stop knowing who you are *without* that validation. Without approval you stop existing.

So instead of just needing others' approval to feel OK, you start to need it to know and be who you are.

I have a very good friend who is a recovered alcoholic. As part of her extensive work sponsoring others going through the Alcoholics Anonymous process, she got a firsthand insight as to why breaking free from alcohol addiction proves so difficult.

At the heart of it was a simple question for recovering alcoholics: Who am I without alcohol?

People with alcohol problems didn't know who they were without alcohol. They didn't know how to handle social situations without a drink, they didn't know how to handle stress without a drink, they didn't know how to just enjoy life without a drink. So, changing no longer simply meant giving up drinking; it meant finding out who they really were. Which felt a lot scarier and so a lot more difficult.

The same question is true for all addictions, including people pleasing. If you are a people pleaser, ask yourself, who are you if you are not pleasing others?

Who are you without that approval? How would you approach your life differently?

IT'S NOT YOUR JOB TO BE EVERYTHING TO EVERYONE

When you're a young child, you know that your survival depends on you being loved and cared for by those around you – your parents, your siblings, your wider family, and whoever is looking after you.

And so, you learn to adapt to what you "need" to be and not be in order to be loved and taken care of. It's a matter of survival.

This makes sense when you're a young child and when you are fully dependent on others to survive. But that very same behavior as an adult is not only not necessary for your survival but will actually create huge problems in your life.

But now it's become learned behavior. And as your social interactions expand far beyond your immediate family, you carry that learned behavior, that "survival mechanism" with you and apply it to nearly every relationship or interaction you have – friendships, work relationships, romantic relationships, any interactions with the world at large.

As you grow and develop into adulthood, you are designed to grow out of dependency into *independence*.

Most people instinctively recognize the obvious elements of this – you no longer need your parents to look after you, to wash you, to feed you, to dress you, to tell you what time to go to bed, and so on. You became independent in all these aspects of your life.

But way, way, way too many people don't fully transition to being *emotionally independent.*

Over time, instead of looking to your parents, teachers, older siblings, etc., for how you should think, how you should behave, and what choices were right and wrong, you are designed to progressively **look to yourself** for these answers – to progressively create and shape your own identity, your own values, your own desires, and your own path through life.

And through developing that independence of thought, that independent sense of your worth and value, you can create a life that makes sense to you, not just to your parents and teachers.

Of course, these choices and your identity is always going to be heavily influenced by your upbringing. But that does not mean you need to be *a hostage* to it.

And foundationally it means that your sense of self, your sense of self-worth, comes from within, not from anyone else or anything external.

And that is why so many people struggle with issues of self-worth.

That is why so many people struggle with a pattern of thinking that they didn't even know they had, that was once a survival mechanism but is no longer necessary; a way of thinking and behaving that they were designed to release in the transition from childhood to adulthood but through bad teaching and parenting (no matter how well intentioned), has remained with them.

But because most people aren't even aware that they are doing it, they adopt this behavior to nearly every relationship. They become a featureless lump of clay, shaped by whomever they come into contact with at any given point in time. They try to be everything to everyone and so *end up being nothing to themselves.*

But that isn't your job and it isn't a worthy goal. You don't exist to make someone else pleased, happy, or OK. That's their job. Just as your job is to be pleased by your own life, by your own choices, and in doing so, be the light for others to do the same.

Until you let go of this way of thinking you cannot create the life or the confidence you desire. Independence of thought, independence of your sense of your own value is essential for your success.

BEFORE YOU ASK WHAT SOMEONE ELSE THINKS OF YOU, ASK YOURSELF WHY YOU CARE

A lion doesn't concern itself with the opinion of sheep

– GEORGE R. R. MARTIN

I'd like you to take a moment and consider how much of your life you spend thinking about what others think of you. Are you thrown off-balance when you hear that someone has criticized you or said something unkind or disrespectful about you?

If so, why?

Why have you chosen to allow the opinion of others to in any way make you feel worse or better about who you are or the choices you make? If your own values and opinions are the highest source of truth (which they are when you have learned to control your mind), why do you allow yourself to think that the opinion of anyone else has a higher value, a higher calling on the truth than your own?

Is this another part of the prison that you, like 99% of the people in the world, have allowed yourself to be trapped in?

Nearly everyone has an opinion about everything these days. No matter who you are or what you do, you can be sure that someone somewhere will criticize you, demean you, belittle you, tell you you're stupid, bad, ugly, wrong, and a million other things as well.

But those opinions are flimsy, transient things that depend far more on what's happening in that person's life and how they are feeling about themselves than on any "reality" about you.

Those opinions are not some God-given statement of truth about who you are and what you've done. So what benefit is there to you in placing any weight on what is said?

If you want the clearest illustration possible of this, take a few moments and log onto YouTube and watch celebrities reading out Mean Tweets on Jimmy Kimmel. Watch those who the world considers to be the most successful, talented, beautiful, wealthiest people on the planet read out some seriously mean, vindictive, and nasty comments.

Think about this for a second: whether or not you like or dislike any individual, you would objectively have to admire the talent and skills that have got them to the place where they are internationally famous and highly successful by any reasonable measure. Yet despite (and in many ways because) of this, they are subject to vile comments and abuse on a daily basis.

Why am I telling you this? I want you to see how foundationless the opinions of other people are. Even when you're in what the world calls the 1%, you will be subject to negativity, criticism, and often abuse.

The foundation of self-confidence is not having your sense of your value, the way you feel about you, determined in any way by other people and external circumstances.

Instead, it is based on your own stable and unshakable view of yourself, no matter what is happening or being said about you.

The answer is for you to know who you are and to focus on what you think of you. That means knowing your values and living in alignment with your values. It means knowing what you want and going after what you want, irrespective of whether all those around you think that is amazing or terrible.

I know my values and my purpose. My values are integrity, kindness, boldness, adventure, growth, and unshakable integrated masculinity. That means that each day I focus on being a better person, a better man, a better father, a better partner, developing my mindset, working on my physical health, and giving my best to the world.

My purpose and my mission is unstoppable self-confidence. I desire to help as many people as possible unleash their natural confidence and success. I desire to free them from the bad teaching and poor programming that holds them back from living the lives they dream of, lives they are entirely capable of living if they simply got out of their own way.

I know my values and my purpose. I know who I am and what I want my life to look like. I have chosen my values carefully after a great deal of consideration. I have chosen my mission with great care and work on it diligently to bring the greatest benefit to myself, to those I love, and to the wider world. I have designed my life in great detail and work on it every day.

I am proud of my values; I am proud of my mission. And I am proud of the way I live my life.

Each and every day I use my values as my "magnetic north" for my decision-making and I live true to my own code for my life and to how I want to behave.

In that context there is nothing anyone could say or do that could ever make me feel bad about who I am or make me feel better about who I am.

As a result, my confidence is completely unshakable.

I know and accept that some people won't like me, what I do, what I say, the choices I make, or how I live. I am completely OK with that. My reference point is not others' opinions but my own values and intuition.

THE MYTH THAT LOVE = SACRIFICE

I want to touch on one of the most deep-rooted and wrong ideas about love that I see almost everywhere.

This idea is that love requires, in fact *it demands,* you to sacrifice yourself in ways big and small; that the act of sacrificing yourself is love.

That the more you sacrifice yourself, the more loving you are; that the degree of sacrifice equates to the depth of love; and that if you don't readily, willingly, joyfully sacrifice yourself then you don't really love the other person.

I could write an entire book on this subject alone, but I think this one way of thinking is responsible for more toxic relationships, for the end of more relationships that could otherwise be strong, vibrant and healthy than almost anything else.

To be clear I am not suggesting that you shouldn't, if required, put yourself in harm's way to protect those you love and care about. I'm not suggesting that relationships don't require negotiation and compromise.

If anyone were to try to harm my children, I wouldn't hesitate to do whatever was necessary, no matter the cost to me, to protect them. The same would be true for my parents, my brother and sister, and for many friends. I would do exactly the same for any partner.

Those are real, noble, and healthy values, and they form part of any relationship.

What I am suggesting is that the idea that love needs, requires, or demands sacrifice is just plain wrong. And that false belief, that bad programming, is why so many relationships fail, causing untold misery.

As I did some research for this part of the book, I came across a (fairly typical) page talking about this subject and I found this quote.

> *"Sacrificing your happiness for the happiness of the one you love is by far the truest type of love. True love is not easy, being in love always demands sacrifice. Sacrifice is the main ingredient in the recipe of love. That's what you do for someone you love...you sacrifice what you feel for whatever they need."*

This quote sums up perfectly the toxic notion that the <u>defining characteristic</u> of love is sacrifice – not something that may be rarely necessary in moments of extreme danger, but something that must be there for love to exist.

That somehow love equals sacrifice and pain.

Now slow down and ask yourself, do you really believe that "true love" involves sacrificing yourself for others? Do you think that your willingness to sacrifice yourself is what makes you a good person, is what demonstrates your love?

Any relationship that demands you sacrifice what matters most to you is a bad relationship. It's not a normal relationship and it's sure as hell not a healthy one.

But most people have this as a foundational belief about love; and it not only destroys your self-esteem and success in life, but it also poisons your personal relationships.

The foundation of all strong, vibrant, healthy relationships isn't sacrifice.

It's respect.

The vital ingredient that makes any successful relationship between any two people is respect, no matter if it is a romantic relationship, a parent-child relationship, a teacher-pupil relationship, a friendship, or a relationship between siblings.

The best relationships are where you have people with strong self-respect, respecting the other person and demanding and requiring respect from others.

Imagine for a moment how different all your relationship would be with this small, simple shift in focus.

The reason this notion of "love equals sacrifice" is so damaging is because when you think you should sacrifice yourself for a relationship, it is an open invitation for others to start disrespecting you.

You start to tolerate bad behavior in your relationships because "true love" demands sacrifice of self. The world has been taught that it requires you to ignore your own value, ignore your own feelings, ignore your pain, and simply accept the bad behavior others may demonstrate in your relationship.

You make "an exception" for the person that you love because they are in a bad mood or have had a bad day, and because you love them you allow yourself to become the target for their bad behavior.

How often do you allow someone "important" to cross your boundaries, to do something you don't like, to behave disrespectfully towards you because you've decided you love them and so must sacrifice yourself for them as well?

Do you realize that when you make these exceptions that you are undoing all the good things you have learned about valuing yourself and treating yourself well?

I'm not suggesting that you have no tolerance for the people you love having good days and bad days or making mistakes. Of course, these things will happen sometimes and they are part of the natural cycle of life and relationships. That's normal, natural, and healthy. But don't ever confuse that with accepting disrespect in the relationship.

If you're honest with yourself, you're fully aware of which people treat you with respect and love but have the normal ups and downs of life, and which people demonstrate a broader pattern of bad behavior.

There's a great quote that says, "The culture of any organization is shaped by the worst behavior the leader is willing to tolerate." Let me rephrase it so it's applicable to you.

Your confidence and success in life is shaped by the worst behavior you are willing to tolerate.

It doesn't matter whether it is a lot of people, a few people, or just one person: when you tolerate bad behavior, you are still telling yourself that you don't matter enough to maintain your self-respect and that you don't expect others to respect you.

If your self-respect is flexible, if it varies according to who you are dealing with, then it doesn't truly exist and you haven't yet seen your true value. You are still sabotaging your own confidence and success for the sake of people who feel OK to treat you badly.

Don't beat yourself up about this if this is you – there's no benefit in that and you should only ever be interested in what benefits you. Be grateful that you've uncovered another bug, another ego trap that would have otherwise kept you stuck for years. Remember that no thought, no decision, stands still. It either helps you or harms you.

So if, for example, you tolerate "just" your partner treating you badly (because you've been taught the lie that true love means sacrifice), it is a cancer to all of your confidence and success.

You won't stand up for yourself because you love the person, and because you love them, you "know" that you're supposed to sacrifice anything and everything for them. And so you're now stuck in a prison – never leaving, simply taking more disrespect and bad treatment to "prove" your love.

Can you see why this is so damaging? It isn't neutral. It isn't some harmless exception that doesn't really matter. It's a decision that will slowly eat away at your self-worth, a mind trap that says you must take the disrespect because "that's what love is." It spills over into other relationships, other situations.

It spreads and spreads because it's just too easy for your ego to find reasons to make evermore exceptions, until there are no exceptions left to make.

And until you've completely lost all respect for yourself and the people around you have lost all respect for you. At which point the relationship is over anyway. Because no one wants a relationship with a door mat.

So why not give up this lie today? Give up on the noxious and entirely *wrong* belief that sacrifice equals love. And instead, retune your thinking just a little so that respect equals love.

You'll be astonished at the results with this simple shift in focus. You'll be astonished at how when you respect yourself, others will respect you too. You'll be astonished by how they start to value and cherish you, and by how you then give all your relationships the chance to work, to make sense, and to be the incredible joy they are meant to be.

And you'll see how your confidence and self-respect naturally starts flowing again from this one simple thought structure.

But for that to happen you need to let go of the bad programming that love equals sacrifice and pain.

So today, why not decide to make this small simple change? Why not stop handing out free passes to people to treat you badly?

OVERCOMING CO-DEPENDENCY

Co-dependency is driven by the agreement that I will work harder on your problem and your life than you do. This is not love.

– KYLO

I want to show you the end game for approval seeking and people pleasing. Unless and until this habit is broken this is where you end up.

The end game is <u>co-dependency</u>. This is, in simple terms, where you come to <u>excessively rely on other people</u> for a sense of approval and a sense of identity. It's when you literally don't know who you are or if you're OK without reference to someone else (usually your partner, but it can be anyone). It happens when you become so invested in a specific relationship you find it hard to function and operate independently.

You may have heard of this term but it's far more widespread than most people understand. On the surface, co-dependency doesn't sound bad. A co-dependent cares about their partner and wants the best for them.

But the issue with co-dependency is that this tips over into having your entire life revolving around your partner. Most of your thoughts and behaviors are centered around your partner. You put aside your own wants, needs, and feelings in order to make sacrifices to please the person that you love.

Overcoming co-dependency is purely about reconnecting with yourself. It's about **unhooking your sense of "being OK" from the reaction, feelings, or actions of your partner**.

It's about detaching from the emotional rollercoaster your partner may be on – their emotions do not define your emotions. You recognize that they are an adult who is responsible for managing their own feelings, as all adults are.

You learn that you are not responsible for other people's problems, issues, circumstances, or behavior. You can show genuine kindness, empathy, and understanding; you can listen with care and attention, but all **without the _need_ to fix things** or make them right.

You cannot love another "better." You can support them, be there for them, and encourage them, but their journey is theirs.

CARE TAKING VS CARE GIVING

Co-dependency is often seen as caretaking and the first question people often ask when they hear this term is "what's wrong with that? Why wouldn't being caring be healthy?"

The reason is that there is a <u>very big difference</u> between caregiving and caretaking. One is healthy, the other is not. Caregiving is rooted in love and kindness. Caretaking is rooted in people pleasing, approval seeking, and insecurity. It is based on **_the need_ _to be needed for fear of loss_**. You cross the line into caretaking when you use your energy and time to handle the problem of someone who is fully capable of handling the problem themselves.

Here are some of the signs you may be caretaking (this is taken from www.therelationshiptherapycenter.com):

• Others often accuse you of crossing personal boundaries, or meddling. But you believe you know what's best for others.

• Other people's ability to take care of themselves seems unlikely.

So, you tend to solve their problems without first giving them the chance to try it themselves.

- Solving other people's problems comes with strings attached, expecting something in return (whether unconscious or not). After all, you sacrificed all your energy and time for them.
- You constantly feel stressed, exhausted, frustrated, and even depressed.
  - Needy people are drawn to you like a magnet.
  - You're often judgmental.
  - You don't take care of yourself because you think that's selfish.

On the other hand, you display **caregiving** when you offer a helping hand to someone who truly needs it. You accept what you can't control and deal with the situation and the person compassionately.

So, caregiving looks very different:

- Well-defined personal boundaries are in place, and you honor those of other people. You believe that you only know what's best for you, not someone else.
- You trust others enough to know that they are capable of solving their own problems. So, you give them a chance to do what they can to handle the issue. You assure them that you're by their side if they need help, but respectfully wait until they ask you to help.
- Instead of keeping account of your good deeds, you give freely of your extra energy and time.
- Giving of yourself feels satisfying, energizing, and even inspirational.
- You don't see the logic in judging others. Instead, you listen and empathize without jumping to conclusions.
- You take care of yourself because you know unless you're healthy and happy you can't give assistance to others.

There is a very big and important difference between being a "nice" person and being genuinely kind because that's just who you are: kind people (as contrasted with "nice" people) have no problem getting into healthy, long-lasting relationships.

Most people who are being nice are doing so because deep down they seek approval. They are seeking to get something (approval, validation, love, being needed) rather than seeking to give something (love, kindness, decency, affection) **without condition**, without the need to get anything in return.

Can you see the difference? Again, most importantly can you <u>feel</u> the difference?

<u>Kindness is going to give; niceness is going to get</u>. Niceness is something unkind disguised as something good – which is why it causes so much confusion. If you are being nice in order to get something in return (even if you are not consciously doing so), then that isn't kind at all. It is a trade, a covert contract that the other person may not want and certainly didn't sign up for.

This is why so many nice people face so much anger and resentment and can't understand why. In their minds, they are being kind. But in truth, they've given their love, niceness, and any otherwise positive acts along with a set of terms and conditions. And then they get pissed off when other people don't meet those unstated terms and conditions.

No one likes niceness with an ulterior motive.

People who are genuinely kind have a strong sense of confidence and are fully comfortable with who they are. They have no problem being kind to others because they value themselves. They give out their love and kindness without any conditions, without any expectation of getting anything in return. They do it because that's simply who they are.

The antidote to co-dependence is self-esteem. Genuinely kind people like themselves and have strong boundaries and strong values. They are not afraid to be strong, assertive, firm, and to say "No" when other people cross the line. They love themselves just as much as they love others, and expect and demand to be treated well.

Kind people don't habitually sacrifice themselves. They like, respect, and love themselves too much for that. And they know that any healthy partner and relationship wouldn't require that.

Kind people are **independent**. That doesn't mean that they don't desire relationships, meaningful, passionate connections with other people. Quite the opposite. But they <u>desire</u> that passion and connection. They don't <u>need</u> it.

They love and cherish their partners and they work at their relationships. But they know that if their relationship ended, they would be OK. Not delighted, not happy, but completely fine. And so that means that they are free to love, to give, and to be kind without condition.

They don't need approval or validation from anyone else. They already give themselves abundant approval and validation.

And because they respect themselves, they attract relationships where their partner respects them, cherishes them, loves them, and gives to them.

And so instead of having a relationship based on sacrifice and getting (directly or indirectly), you have a relationship based on respect, kindness, love, and giving.

A healthy relationship.

Which all flows from their own self-esteem, respect, and confidence. This means they have no requirement whatsoever to please others, to seek the approval of others, or to be validated in any way by others.

LIVE LIFE TRUE TO YOURSELF

Do you know the number one regret people have on their deathbed?

Consistently, the single biggest regret of people at the end of their lives is that they wish they'd had the courage to live a life true to themselves, instead of the life that others expected of them.

They wish they'd truly gone after their dreams instead of settling for what only seemed like a safe and comfortable existence.

They wish they'd honored their own choices instead of the ones they felt they should.

They wish they'd taken the risk to live their best life instead of playing safe and small.

They wish they'd ignored the lies of those around them trying to "help" them, who said that it "can't be done," that it doesn't happen for people "like you," to get realistic.

They wish they'd taken all the opportunities that they can now see that life put right in front of them – opportunities that they let their fears and their desire to please others block them from.

The tragedy is that most people only realize this when it's genuinely too late, on their deathbed and there is no more time to change. Finally, only when their life draws to a close do they see the truth that was always there.

The truth that at any point they could have made different choices, authentic choices, the choices that really made sense for them to be who they wanted to be and to live the life they wanted to live.

To not waste their precious lives in a destructive attempt to please another, when all they ever had to do was learn to please themselves first.

That choice is right in front of you today, in all kinds of ways big and small. All you need to do is observe, *not judge*, the ways in which you may be trying to please those around you.

The simple act of observing your behavior, thoughts, and feelings, and observing whether people pleasing helps you or harms you is all you need to start to break free from this mental prison.

The door to the prison is open. It always was and it always will be. But you have to choose to walk through it.

I can show you the way out and everything you need to live an incredible life outside in the real world. But ultimately the choice is always yours.

Most people don't give themselves that choice until it's too late.

So today, why not think about, and then go and live free of the need to please others? Why not live free of the need to bend yourself out of shape to fit in? Why not just be you?

You might find you like it. And you will absolutely find that it's the path to your confidence and success.

THINGS TO CONSIDER

- Can you see that being a people pleaser means that you become other people's prisoner, their servant? Is this something you would consciously choose? Are you happy to choose it consciously or unconsciously?

- Can you see that people pleasing means that you are choosing to make what other people think more important than what you think? That your thoughts, your desires, your needs, your choices, and your values matter less?

- Consider that being a people pleaser makes you inauthentic and dishonest about who you really are and what you really think and feel. How do you feel about continuing to be inauthentic and dishonest? Don't feel bad, just consider this.

- Consider that people pleasing isn't kind behavior at all. It is giving with an ulterior motive. It is a trade (that the other person never signed up for) where you behave in inauthentic ways to get their approval.

- Consider that until you give up people pleasing, you can never get the life you dream of.

- Consider: Have you allowed yourself to be emotionally dependent on others in order to feel OK about who you are? If so, don't feel bad (there is no benefit in that). Instead, just consider if you want this to continue.

- Consider for a moment the empowering truth that no matter who you are and no matter what you do, some people will like, love, and approve of you and some won't. Knowing that, no matter what, some people will disapprove of you, consider if there are actually any benefits to people pleasing.

- What would your life look like if you gave up any need to please others and instead focused on approving of yourself?

- Have you fallen for the myth that love equals sacrifice?

- Consider that the basis for all great relationships isn't sacrifice but respect.

- Consider: Does people pleasing have any place in your life from now on?

THE MAGIC OF MAKING MISTAKES

When a child learns to walk and falls down 50 times, they never think to themselves "maybe this isn't for me."

ANONYMOUS

W hat does "failure" mean to you?

How do you *feel* (not think) about what the world calls failure? How do you feel when you make a mistake, when you fail at something?

By looking at how you feel instead of how you think, you tune into the real meaning that "failure" has for you. And that's where you need to dig, to find the buried thought patterns that sabotage you without you knowing it.

You've likely read lots of motivational quotes on what failure "ought to mean," but as I've said previously, reading something, intellectually knowing it and understanding it, <u>is very different from living it</u> as a way of life. Only when you live it as a way of life do you truly know something.

Take a few moments now and feel what failure means to you. Remember that this is only for your benefit so be honest.

Here are a few questions for you:

- Do you feel good or bad when you think about failure?
- Do you look forward to failing more or is it something you secretly dread even if you know you "shouldn't"?
- Do you think of failure as something you are or something you do? Or maybe both? Be honest with yourself here. This is to help you.
- Do you see failure as an event or as a process?

Give yourself a few minutes to consider these questions and take a note of the answers.

So, did you do it? Or did your ego get you to just skip past that bit and tell you you'd get around to doing it later? Remember that the change you want requires you to do more than simply read – it comes from considering and applying. There are no extra bonus points for getting to the end of the book the quickest. The challenge isn't being the first to read to the end; the challenge is to get the greatest benefit.

CHANGING THE MEANING OF FAILURE

Our greatest glory is not in never falling, but in rising every time we fall.

– CONFUCIUS

Most people, if they were honest, don't like failing. They feel bad when they fail and believe that the act of failing reveals some kind of shortcoming within them.

In an earlier chapter I talked about the difference between a fixed mindset and a growth mindset. It may not surprise you to know that the majority of people have a fixed mindset. And those with a fixed mindset view failure differently and in a far more negative, damaging, and sabotaging way than those with a growth mindset.

If you have a fixed mindset, you believe your talents and capabilities are fixed and unchanging. You see every single test, every single attempt to do pretty much anything as a means by which those fixed talents and capabilities are *revealed*.

Any failure then reveals the underlying "truth" that they are in some way not good enough, talented enough, or capable enough.

The fixed mindset turns failure into a verdict on who you are, your value, on your *innate* ability to become who you want to be and to create the life you want to live.

This means that failure can be deeply wounding, even traumatic – because why would you look forward to the possibility of having an unchangeable shortcoming, an inherent flaw or deficiency exposed and confirmed?

Each time you took on a challenge it is no longer simply a matter of how the challenge goes, *but how you measure up.* Forever. Full stop.

And each time you fall short of the perceived standard, or fare less well than others, it is another door closed, another possibility turned into a dead end.

It is this way of thinking that turns failure from being something you do into something that you are.

It is why so many people have such a deep-rooted fear of failure. Each failure represents a "confirmed" narrowing of your horizons, a definitive reduction in the possibilities for your life, a black mark against your name for some shortcoming without any possibility of redemption.

With that kind of thinking, there is no upside to risking failure. And so, it's better for it to be avoided altogether – which is exactly what you may have noticed that most people do.

The problem goes further though.

How you feel about failure defines how you respond to failure, how you respond to any setbacks in life. Because if you see a failure as a definitive (negative) verdict on your talents and who you are, why bother even responding? After all, you already have your answer.

In her book *Mindset*, Carol Dweck refers to a study of seventh graders who were asked how they would respond to an academic failure (a poor test grade on a course).

Those with the growth mindset said they would study harder for the next test. But those with the fixed mindset said they would *study less* for the next test.

Why?

Well, the thinking of those with fixed mindsets was that if you already "know" you don't have the ability, why waste your time? They also said they would seriously consider cheating! If you don't have the ability, they thought, you just have to look for another way.

Dweck reveals how their response also limits the future life chances of those with a fixed mindset. Instead of trying to learn from and address the lessons of their failure, people with a fixed mindset may simply try to repair their self-esteem in a destructive way.

She cites the example of college students who, after doing poorly on a test, were given the chance to look at the tests of the other students. Those with a growth mindset looked at the tests of those who had done far better than they had. They wanted to learn from their failure. They wanted to learn the lessons so that they could get better, stronger, and wiser.

But students with the fixed mindset chose instead to look at the tests of those who had done *really poorly*. Why? Because if they could find people who had done much worse than them, if those results were also facts, then they felt better about themselves because *they were not as bad as someone else*.

This action didn't improve their own opportunities for future success. It simply acted as confirmation that others were worse. And so instead of looking to break the glass ceiling above them, which they now accepted as fixed and immovable, they focused instead on building an unstable foundation beneath them to shore up their self-image.

This was based on "not being as bad as" rather than on "how good could I become?"

Based on that response, based on the decision to focus on shoring up their self-esteem instead of on their learning and growth, those *perceived limits* transformed into facts, backed up by "real" evidence.

There was nothing inherently true about their perceived inability to improve, but their perceptions and mindsets *made it true*.

TURNING FAILURE INTO HELPLESSNESS

Here's where this gets really damaging. Over time, this way of thinking, this lens on your sense of who you are as a fixed set of talents, pre-programmed at birth, sets you up for learned helplessness.

If you feel that in any given area you either have a winning or losing lottery ticket, you create a sense that you only have control over your life in a very limited way. Those areas where you are "good" only remain good until you make a mistake. And as soon as you make a mistake, then even your sense of being good in that area becomes shaky and unstable.

Each new set of challenges and results can only either confirm what you already knew or undermine your sense of your talents if you don't perform to an acceptable standard. There is no upside, only the risk of "taking away" what you already have.

Consider for a moment what this way of thinking does to your chances of creating success. Remember, as my friend Andy Shaw taught me, no thought is neutral. Every thought either helps you or harms you.

The thought that your talents are fixed, set in stone, and unchangeable works against your ability to grow, to change, and to become more. It only takes a single failure to close the door on a whole area of your life, a whole set of opportunities that could otherwise lead to your highest good.

With that way of thinking, a single mistake is all that is ever needed to reduce your life chances. In this way of thinking, you've either won the genetic lottery or you didn't, so why bother trying?

With a fixed mindset, you set yourself up to always be measured by failure, never by success. Failures anchor people with a fixed mindset to the ground <u>and leaves them no route to success</u>.

If they fail at something they feel less worthy, less deserving...just less. And the more they feel this way, the less action they take to solve their problems.

And so, a negative spiral is created. In fact, as Carol Dweck points out:

"In short when people believe in fixed traits, they are always in danger of being measured by failure. It can define them in a permanent way. Smart or talented as they may be, this mindset seems to rob them of their coping resources."

But science has proven that in every meaningful sense your traits are <u>not fixed</u>. They are entirely adaptable, moldable, and can be shaped by the right thoughts and actions.

NEUROPLASTICITY

I want to take a slight detour for a moment to talk you through the concept of brain plasticity or what's now called neuroplasticity. This is so you grasp just how powerful your brain really is, and, more importantly, how the entire sense that your talents and capabilities are fixed has been scientifically proven to be false. For this section I've called on articles by Dr. Pascale Michelon and Dr. Majid Fotuhi.

The scientifically proven truth that your capabilities are not fixed in any way matters, because the limits most people place on themselves are based on false assumptions and false facts. By shattering these lies, by showing how clearly and scientifically wrong these sabotaging beliefs are, you can set yourself free and begin to unleash your nearly limitless potential.

Neuroplasticity refers to the brain's (by which I mean the physical organ of your brain as opposed to your mind) ability to change throughout life.

For a long time, science believed that as we aged, the connections in the brain became fixed and locked into place. This meant that, for a long time, science also believed that your capabilities were largely fixed.

However, more recent research has shown that to be false. In fact, it's now recognized that the brain (the actual physical, organic tissue) has an amazing ability to reorganize itself by forming new connections between brain cells (neurons), to reshape itself in response to stimuli.

In addition to genetic factors, the environment in which you live, as well as your thoughts and actions all play a substantial role in shaping your brain.

Neuroplasticity occurs in the brain:

1) At the beginning of life when the immature brain organizes itself for the first time.

2) In the case of brain injury, to compensate for lost functions or to maximize remaining functions.

3) Through adulthood whenever something new is learned.

There are a few striking examples of this that bring this concept to light. Research has shown that London taxi drivers have a larger hippocampus (in the posterior region) than London bus drivers.

Why is that?

Because this region of the hippocampus specializes in acquiring and using complex spatial information in order to navigate efficiently. Taxi drivers have to navigate around London whereas bus drivers simply follow a limited set of predefined routes.

Those who are bilingual also show changes in brain anatomy. Learning a second language is possible through *functional* changes in the brain;

the left inferior parietal cortex is larger in bilingual brains than in monolingual brains.

Neuroplasticity was also seen in the brains of musicians compared to non-musicians. Studies showed cortex volume was highest in professional musicians, intermediate in amateur musicians, and lowest in non-musicians in several brain areas involved in playing music: motor regions, anterior superior parietal areas, and inferior temporal areas.

There has also been clear research to show that extensive learning of new information can also trigger plastic changes in the brain. One study imaged the brains of medical students three months before their medical exam and right after the exam, and compared them to the brains of students who were not studying for exams at that time.

The medical students' brains showed learning induced changes in the regions of the parietal cortex and the posterior hippocampus, which are the regions known to be involved in memory retrieval and learning.

There are even incredible stories of how certain functions can move from one area of the brain to another in response to brain injury. The brain literally rewires itself to maximize function after injury.

You don't need to understand all the technical language, *but simply to understand the astonishing truth.*

The human brain, <u>your brain</u>, adapts and physically changes to support you mastering the skills, the information, and the ways of thinking and acting that best serve the <u>primary activities</u> in your life.

Your brain is essentially no different to a muscle. ***<u>In the same way that you can strengthen your body through exercise, so too can you strengthen your mind.</u>***

Can you grasp what this means for you, for your life? For your ability to learn, develop, grow, and master anything you desire? Your brain will <u>physically adapt</u> for you to master anything you focus on. It will literally reshape itself to optimize the skills and knowledge you choose to master and which are your dominant focus in life.

It is designed to support mastery of whatever skills and information you need at any given point in time.

Can you see now the fallacy of how most of the world views failure?

THE NATURAL PROCESS OF SUCCESS

Every failure is a lesson. If you are not willing to fail,
you are not ready to succeed.

– KEN ROBINSON

How you truly feel about failure (rather than what you think you should feel about it) defines how far you will go in creating the life you desire.

Most of the world has read countless quotes on the value of failure, but not 1 in 100 people come close to applying it and even fewer live it as a way of life. So, the reading of the quotes, the posting of them on social media, only gives the illusion of progress.

And it means that most people never understand what the quotes really mean in the first place.

So, if, for example, you **knew** that every failure is a lesson, if you knew that failure made you stronger, wiser, better equipped to ultimately succeed, why would you fear it?

If you did know this you, would <u>run towards failure</u>; you would be happy (even delighted) to fail and have no fear of it at all, merely **respect for the benefits it gives you**.

You would understand that mastery in any area can only be achieved through failure. You would understand the foolishness of people telling you that "failure is not an option" and would instead know that not only is failure an option, but it is often the best option.

Failing is the way we are designed to learn and grow.

Let me repeat that: <u>failure is the way we are designed to learn and grow</u>.

Failure is the natural process of success and mastery.

Here's how you are designed to learn, grow, and achieve anything in your life:

- You decide something you want to be, do, or have.
- You take steps towards that goal.
- You fail.
- You (quickly or slowly) understand the lessons that you need to apply to get better and to make progress.
- You learn (by which I mean, apply) these lessons.
- Rinse and repeat.
- You keep going <u>until</u> you reach your goal.

Whether you realize it or not, this is how you've learned everything you currently know, how you've acquired every skill you currently have, and how you've achieved every goal you've ever completed.

Each failure was a lesson to give you precisely the experience, tools, wisdom, and learning that you needed to get the outcome you desired.

Without that learning, the goals wouldn't have been possible. You needed that data, that feedback, that experience to become better, stronger, and wiser. Failure was essential to your success (and remember that essential means "cannot happen without").

You were at your most successful during the first few years of your life. You learned more, developed more, and achieved more at this stage in your life than at any other.

You learned to crawl, walk, talk, socially interact, play, feed yourself, laugh, smile, explore, and problem-solve for the first time.

And you failed more times in these first few years than at any other time in your life. <u>Does that mean you were a failure? Or did you simply follow the natural process of learning more than at any other time</u>?

Was it before you were programmed with any (false) sense that your talents and capabilities were fixed? Imagine the madness of a young child learning to walk and failing a test and then thinking that the test revealed that they were incapable of walking?

Do they fall over (fail) countless times in the process of learning? Do they sometimes get bumps and bruises as they learn control of their bodies and find out the best ways to sit up, get on their knees, push themselves up, balance themselves, put one foot in front of the other while holding on, and then eventually simply walk?

Do they make the most progress by being taught to walk in a classroom or by following the natural model of learning?

Once again, it is bad teaching that takes us away from the way we are designed to live, learn, and grow. By applying false and negative meaning to things that are there to help us, <u>we block the very means by which we achieve the success we desire</u>.

Those who are masters of anything – business, sport, dating, mindset, etc. – *only achieved that position of mastery* through experiencing more failures than 99% of people would even attempt.

Don't just read that quickly: slow down and think about it.

Michael Jordan, arguably the greatest basketball player of all time, once said:

> *"I've missed more than 9,000 shots in my career. I've lost almost 300 games. Twenty-six times I've been trusted to take the game-winning shot and missed. I've failed over and over and over again in my life. And that is why I succeed."*

If you look at nearly any successful person, I pretty much guarantee that they will have experienced more failures, got more things wrong, made more mistakes, and taken more wrong turns than everyone else.

The fear of failure is simply the adult version of monsters under the bed. But in this case, not only is the monster not there, your hidden treasure is there instead. Through inaccurate and wrong beliefs about the meaning of failure, that treasure stays hidden away, locked beneath the bed for fear of even looking.

Failure, despite how nearly the whole world sees it, is your very best friend.

So why do so many people cling to a belief that the evidence overwhelmingly shows is false?

There is a massive difference between how the 1% see failure, and the 99% who want to succeed but never take the actions necessary to create the success that they are capable of.

The 1% know that they will ultimately succeed and so they embrace the journey (the failures) to get there. They do not fear failure because they *know*, they have removed all doubt, **that their success is certain**. So, failure is simply part of the journey, never the end of the journey. They relax and are able to embrace their failures, to squeeze out every bit of value from them because that simply speeds them on their journey to *inevitable* success.

When you know your success is inevitable, what do you have to fear?

Each step along the journey is one where you either win (learn a lesson from a failure) or win big (get the result you desire). Either way, you win. And you don't just win in a specific sense, but in a general one, because you go forward with skills you didn't previously have, with experience you hadn't previously gained, and with knowledge and wisdom you weren't previously aware of that you can apply in all areas of your life. And you have the momentum of getting stronger with each "failure."

The 99% really want to succeed and might even intellectually understand that they will probably experience some failure along the way. But they are secretly scared that they will ultimately fail; they doubt their ultimate success and so they avoid failure as if their lives depend on it.

The irony and tragedy is that it is the avoidance of failure (as a process, as part of the journey) that causes them to ultimately fail – because they never give themselves the chance to learn the required lessons and become the person they need to be to achieve the outcome they desire.

Can you see this difference? When you know your success is certain, your journey becomes enjoyable and you can embrace your failures because you know the outcome is positive. Conversely, if you doubt the outcome, you are sabotaging your success before you even get started because you set yourself up to experience the failure that you need in order to achieve the success you desire.

THE NEXT STEP – FAILURE REVEALS YOUR PATH TO GREATER SUCCESS

Failure is simply the opportunity to begin again, more intelligently.

– HENRY FORD

The benefits of failure stretch well beyond the immediate lessons you need to achieve your specific desired outcome. Failure on a much bigger scale often yields much bigger benefits, some quite staggeringly so.

If you look at the histories of the most successful people, you will see how their greatest failures led directly to their greatest successes – how they never would have been able to create the incredible success they did without the failures they experienced along the way. In fact, most of them credit their litany of failures as the foundation upon which their success was built.

Failure revealed new paths, new possibilities, new opportunities that never would have seemed possible without the failure.

Winston Churchill is now widely regarded as the greatest prime minister the United Kingdom has ever had. He won the Nobel Prize, and when the UK stood largely alone against the Nazis in World War Two, it was Churchill's brilliance, steadfast determination, and utter refusal to yield that prevented Hitler sweeping all of Europe before him. There is now even a statue of Churchill in the Oval Office such is the recognition of his bravery and significance in defeating Nazism.

Much less well known is the fact that Churchill lost <u>every single election</u> he ran in for political office until he became prime minister at the age of 62. He had faced multiple military defeats, some calamitous when he was in the army.

Consider for a moment what Churchill learned from facing these failures – how much stronger, wiser, and more experienced he was to face down the overwhelming odds of defeat in World War Two having experienced and come through all those previous failures. Do you think Churchill's famous indomitable spirit, his unshakable confidence in his path, was helped or harmed by his history of failure?

Do you think that he was given exactly the experiences he needed, exactly when he needed them to prepare him for his eventual greatest success? Do you think he could have achieved that success without having experienced the failure?

Abraham Lincoln is equally widely regarded as one of the greatest US presidents. He is repeatedly cited by serving presidents as their inspiration and role model. What he achieved while in office is staggering.

Yet like Churchill, his life prior to becoming president was littered with setbacks and failures. He failed in business twice, was made bankrupt, and he lost nine elections for public office. His fiancé died and he suffered a nervous breakdown.

Do you think Lincoln's astonishingly clear-sighted and calm leadership, his ability to unite the country after the Civil War, his decision to end slavery in the US, would have been possible without the setbacks and failures he previously experienced?

Can you see the importance of failure, when you look at all the available evidence that failure is an essential ingredient for your ultimate success?

Let me repeat that so you don't miss the importance of what's being said.

Failure is an essential ingredient for your ultimate success.

Failure can and will lead to your greatest success if instead of seeing it as a problem that defines you, you see it as an experience to be faced, dealt with, and learned from.

Carol Dweck uses a brilliant example to illustrate this. She tells the story of Jim Marshall, a former defensive player for the Minnesota Vikings. In a game against the San Francisco 49ers, Marshall saw the football on the ground, picked it up, and ran for a touchdown. To his horror he realized that he had run the wrong way and had scored for the opposition team. On national television. He was devastated.

He had the choice then of being <u>defined by that failure</u> or <u>using that failure</u> as an opportunity to learn, grow, and reach levels that he never would have attained without that experience.

He chose the latter instead of, as he put it, "sitting in my misery." In the second half, he played some of his best football ever and contributed to his team's victory.

But that isn't actually the most important part of the story. As a result of what happened, he spoke to groups of people dealing with failure. He answered letters that poured into him from people who could now relate to him, sharing their own experiences of failure and embarrassment. He focused on improving his concentration during games. He used the experience to become a better player and a better person.

The experience did define him <u>but in empowering ways</u>, in ways that expanded his life, his horizons, his experiences, and his ability to help others. In short, he used his failure in the way he (and you) are naturally designed to use it.

Because of his choice to **use failure,** to leverage it for future success, rather than **be defined by failure**, he became a greater success and in far more wide-reaching ways than ever would have been possible without the failure. He touched more lives, helped more people, inspired more change than would have been previously possible.

He could not have succeeded without that failure. The success (helping huge numbers of people) could never have existed without the failure, so the failure was **necessary**.

MY OWN STORY OF FAILURE

I struggled with a fear of failure for many years, but through experiencing some of the biggest failures of my life and through seeing firsthand the benefits of those failures, I not only overcame my fear but came to see failure for what it really is.

Failure is not an enemy to be feared, but my very best teacher and friend. *It's not something that takes things away from me but something that gives to me in abundance.* Sometimes, though, the abundance is disguised as lack.

Several years ago, I decided to start my own business. I found a business idea that I really liked, one that I knew could be successful and make money. I had always done well academically and had read plenty of business and self-help books and so felt I was ready. I refinanced my home for some start-up investment in the business, quit my job, and set off to work on it.

A year and a half later, I had burned through all the money but I still hadn't even launched the business. It remained nothing more than an idea. I felt embarrassed, humiliated, and a complete failure. I mean, I hadn't even launched the business! I had to set out to find a new job with a gaping hole on my CV and nothing to show for it.

To most people, I had failed and in a pretty laughable way – to not even launch the business was some achievement.

But I quickly realized two of the most important lessons I have ever learned. First, no one else really cared that much that I had failed. It was a big deal to me at the time, but it was of no significance at all to them. They weren't embarrassed for me; they didn't think I had failed (at least not in the way that I did at the time). In fact, the most frequent comment I got was how brave I was for going for it.

In my first interview for a job after giving up on the business, I was concerned how I would justify the 18-month gap on my CV and what impact that would have on my ability to get a job and earn what I had previously earned. So, the question came up and I explained that I had tried to start a business but it had failed.

Their response? They simply said, "Good for you, well done for having the balls to go for it." I got the job, earning substantially more money than I had previously.

That response blew me away. The realization just dropped on me that I had feared for months how I would face people after failing, what they would think of me, how I would deal with the embarrassment. But that wasn't anyone else's response. Only my own.

My fear of failure was in every conceivable way an invention; the things I laid in bed at night thinking about never got any further than my head. They weren't real. I saw that I had caused myself incredible pain, fear, and anguish because of <u>stories I had decided would be true</u>.

Can you imagine the freedom I felt (and that you would feel) having experienced just how baseless my fear of failure was? I saw firsthand that these fears had been a complete and total waste of time and they had simply gotten in the way of me calling time on the business much sooner.

My fear of failure had turned a quick failure into a long failure.

Second, because I had experienced the challenges of starting a business, of raising money and selling my business idea to investors (and despite being told endlessly that I would struggle to do this, it wasn't that hard), I quickly realized that I had experience that massively increased my skills, experience, expertise, and authority in ways I could not have previously conceived. I had learned the critical lessons of how to start a business and how not to, what mattered and what didn't.

Immediately after starting my job, I used all of those skills and experience to develop a new business on the side, one that I could run while doing my job; I made a lot more money a lot more quickly, with a lot less risk and hassle than I could have previously achieved. I made back the money I had put into the first business very quickly.

All of this resulted directly from my failure.

Let me give you one other example in a different part of life. My marriage was a failure. Both my ex-wife and I made numerous mistakes, multiple wrong turns, and didn't make each other happy.

At the end of my marriage, I had completely lost myself trying to hold our family together, giving up more and more of who I was, what made me the person I was, what mattered most to me – my values and my self-respect. I didn't like or respect myself by the end of it. I didn't even know who I was at the end. Family and friends could see that it was an unhappy situation.

So, my marriage failed and I felt like a complete failure; not just as a husband, but as a man, and as an individual. I felt that I was failing my children. And financially, as most people who have been through a divorce will tell you, it is pretty devastating.

But as backwards as it might sound, no experience, nothing, has been as profoundly transformative and rewarding as my divorce. Not only do I not regret my divorce, I am filled with a deep gratitude for having had that experience.

Through my divorce I received the greatest gifts I have ever been given. First, I learned (because I had to) how to get back in control of my mind. I learned this so well that it has never fallen away. As soon as I have any bad feelings at all now, I realize that I have lost control of my mind for a moment.

But I now have exactly the tools and techniques to regain control quickly and easily.

And because I used them, tested them, and proved them in the white heat of a divorce battle, I know just how powerful they are.

Second, I connected with two people who have profoundly impacted and benefitted my life, the two people who were the core inspiration for the material in this book: Andy Shaw and Stephen Hedger.

They showed me the path, the secrets to anyone living as the person they want to be (and really are), and creating the life they want to live. Their teaching, the wisdom they both shared with me through the divorce process and through helping me rebuild my life, has been the most incredible gift I can imagine.

And that is the gift I am sharing with you in this book.

Without that experience, there is no way I would have learned what I now know; there is no way I could have created the life I have now; and there is no way my mind would be as it is now.

Lastly, by <u>using my failure</u> instead of being <u>defined by my failure</u>, I found my life purpose, teaching the world one mind at a time how to unleash the natural confidence and success mindset that we are all born with.

I had been searching for this sense of purpose all my life, wondering whether I would ever find the calling that would unleash all the talents and passion that I knew were within me.

Not only did it show me my path, it put in my path the perfect two mentors – to teach me at exactly the right time, in exactly the right way, exactly what I needed to learn.

I have had the joy of teaching this way of thinking to my two beautiful, incredible daughters and watching them learn these mindsets and flourish as a result has been one of the most wonderful, rewarding experiences of my life.

I get numerous messages each week from people thanking me for how I have helped them, set them free, and changed their lives in all kinds of ways big and small – all through doing something that I love.

Can you see how incredible the gifts that failure has given me are?

There is no amount of money you could offer me to turn back the clock and change any of that experience. That is how valuable the experience has been.

So why on earth would you fear failure?

I want to really lay this out for you so you can understand how backwards and destructive a fear of failure is to your being able to live the life you desire.

The biggest leaps forward in my own life have come directly from my biggest failures. Every success I have created has its roots in a previous failure.

My two biggest failures have taught me more, given me more, developed me more, and sped me on my journey more than any success **ever** has.

Each failure brought with it the wisdom of realizing that failure was not only nothing to fear but something to embrace – something through which the greatest gifts of my life are received. I didn't just read that in a book; I experienced it, I lived it, and so now I know it and live it as a way of life.

It is almost impossible now for me to fear failure, because I simply know that I will either get what I desire, or I will get an incredible lesson that opens the door to something far bigger. So, I either win or I win big.

Without failure, there is no way that I ever could have understood this, ever could have experienced so much incredible joy, richness, and abundance. So, the only thing I remain truly conscious of is *giving myself enough opportunity to fail*.

Consider: Could you choose to look at your failures as your opportunity to begin again more intelligently?

Can you look back at your own failures and see the lessons you were being given? Even if you couldn't see them at the time, can you now see the gifts life was offering you?

Take a little time with this. The gifts are there, I guarantee it. You only need to slow down for long enough to consider what they are, or what they could be.

Don't feel bad if you did miss them; there is no benefit in that and it is simply a mind trap that your ego uses to keep you stuck. Instead, be delighted that you can now see the lessons, that you are now aware enough to look for the lessons. Remember not 1 in 100 people ever learn to do this, so you're already way ahead.

Consider now that the only way to truly fail is to decide that you are a failure, to not learn the lessons.

WHAT IF PLAYING IT SAFE IS THE BIGGEST RISK OF ALL?

Some failure in life is inevitable. It is impossible to live without failing at something, unless you live so cautiously that you might as well not have lived at all – in which case you fail by default.

– J K ROWLING

Has a fear of failure stopped you from going after your dreams?

Have you, like most of the world, chosen to avoid the fear of the unknown and remain in suffering that is familiar?

Most people completely misunderstand the risks they are taking. They focus on the <u>prevention of risk</u>. Maybe this is you too. But have you ever really stopped, slowed down long enough to consider whether this is right? Because it has become an almost unquestionable truth that preventing, stopping, or blocking risks is a good thing, most people have stopped looking at it.

So many of our challenges come from judgement instead of observation. The problem is once you make a decision, a judgement, all thinking stops. Before you make a judgement, you look at things, consider things, evaluate things. Your mind is open to seeing all the possibilities and options instead of just some of them.

But once that decision is made, whether you are conscious of that decision being made or not, your thinking in that area shuts down.

Most people will say that they assess risk and make an informed decision. But ask yourself if this is really true. And if it was true, would there be plenty of occasions where people took the risk instead of the safe option?

Isn't the reality for most people that they default to what they perceive to be the least risky, the safest option pretty much every time? This is where you have to be careful of the words that people use and look at the actions taken instead – **because it is people's actions that reveal their true thinking, not their words**.

The truth is that when most people, the 99%, "assess risk," the real meaning is that they fear risks and want to stop, block, or, at the very least, minimize them.

Their focus is almost entirely on the avoidance of pain or loss and almost never on what they could gain.

But what if that decision isn't actually the way to minimize the risks for your life? What if, by constantly seeking to minimize risk (or perhaps more accurately, the perceived risk), you are actually increasing the overall risks to your life?

What if you are minimizing the opportunities for your life, not just the risks? How often does that form part of the risk assessment being undertaken?

The 1% consider (and I mean, really consider) <u>**both the opportunity arising from the risk and the downside**</u>. They look at the loss of the opportunity by not taking the risk as much as they look at any potential risk of taking action.

As I've said, the problem is that most people completely misjudge and misunderstand the risks that they are taking.

They think that taking the chance is what puts them at risk, **which means that they <u>only look at the downsides</u> of taking the risk**. The mental assessment they make is "If I don't do anything, I keep (don't lose) what I already have. What do I risk losing if I do take action?"

But the 1% who create the life of their dreams make a different assessment. It is the one the 99% think they are making but in reality, are not. And in that difference lies one of the biggest reasons so few people create the life they want and never truly become the person they want to be.

The mental risk assessment the 1% make is, "What do I have to gain from taking this risk? What new possibilities and opportunities will be open and available to me from taking action? What will I learn from taking this action even if it doesn't work out? How can I mitigate the possible risks from taking this action and still get most (or all) of the benefit?"

Can you see the difference? More importantly, can you feel the difference?

Can you see how the assessment of the 1% is focused on the upside, about how they can make progress while dealing with any risks? Conversely, the 99% focus on the risk of loss and the downsides of taking action.

They never truly consider the downsides of doing nothing. They misunderstand that <u>focusing on protection instead of growth</u> creates the certainty of never achieving their dreams, of never becoming all that they could be, of never experiencing the abundance of life available to them. So, they live a stunted, half-baked version of life.

They think they have protected themselves from failure, disappointment, and loss. In reality, though, they have created exactly that failure, disappointment, and loss as a certainty and on a much bigger scale by playing small and staying in suffering merely disguised as safety and comfort.

THE "SAFE PROBLEM"

I see many people remain in situations they know are unhappy, negative, or sometimes even toxic because they fear the risks of change: maybe it's a job with a bad culture; maybe it's staying single because you fear being vulnerable; maybe it's staying in a bad relationship because you fear you won't find someone else to be with or to love you.

What are you allowing in your life that you no longer should? What negative situations, toxic people, bad behavior, intolerance, disrespect, and unhappiness are you allowing to continue in your life?

It's called the "safe problem."

Your ego continually throws fears, doubts, and anxieties at you to keep you stuck and to keep you playing small. It does this by taking something bad (tolerating bad situations or behavior) and presenting it as something good (by telling you that you're safe enough here and the new situation or circumstances might be dangerous).

The problem is that almost no one questions whether this is really true and whether this really does keep you safe.

In fact, all it usually does is keep you miserable, keep you stuck, and sabotage your chances of success and happiness.

And that doesn't keep you safe at all.

For example, way, way, way too many people tolerate disrespect in their personal relationships. They allow their partner to treat them badly in ways big and small. They tolerate the behavior because they fear that if they confront it, it will cause the end of the relationship. But this is complete and total nonsense and it's incredibly damaging and toxic thinking.

The more you tolerate disrespect, the worse it will become. It categorically will not get better. Soon enough the disrespect becomes contempt and study after study will show you that a relationship (in any meaningful sense) is dead once one partner feels contempt for the other.

So, despite the lies your ego has told you, you haven't stayed safe. You've actually brought about the very scenario you were trying to protect yourself from.

And in the process, you've sabotaged your own self-esteem. And you've wasted your time with someone disrespectful instead of giving yourself the opportunity to find someone who will treat you in the ways that you deserve.

None of that sounds like you're being kept safe in any way **at all**.

Today, spend a little time looking at what you are tolerating. Consider whether it's really keeping you safe or actually leading you away from becoming the person you want to be and living the life you want to live.

HOW TO REMOVE THE FEAR OF RISK

To live like the 1%, to create the life you want, and to become the confident successful person you want to be, you have to see risk and failure differently from the 99%.

This doesn't mean taking crazy risks. It does mean <u>looking at risks accurately</u> and taking calculated, informed, and **intelligent risks**. It means seeing that more often than not, the real risk lies in not moving forward and that playing it safe usually means risking staying stuck and not gaining anything.

I want to show you a technique that Andy showed me to unblock myself anytime I realized I was playing it safe.

The key is to see risk accurately, as something that gives you the possibility to win and move forward rather than something you stand to lose from. To do this, take any specific risk you're looking at.

Then go and visit in your mind the best-case scenario, the worst-case scenario, and the scenario where you don't take the risk. See all three scenarios happening in your mind. Look at them in detail. Allow yourself to really go and explore all the things that could happen. Look at the very best and the very worst things you can see happening in each scenario.

Remember, you are just exploring this in your mind, so it's completely safe. There is nothing to fear – you are just looking.

Once you've done this, explore and consider all the ways you **win no matter what**. Yes, all the ways you win if things go well and all the ways you win if it "goes wrong," and all the ways you win if you decide that this isn't the right choice for you.

See all the benefits, all the things you gain from the best-case scenario happening: see and feel how much closer you are to creating the life you desire; how happy and pleased you are that you overcame your fears and moved forward; how you stopped being a prisoner to a false view of risk; how you now move forward with greater ease; and how you've expanded your ability to create what you want in your life.

See all the benefits from it going completely wrong in the worst-case scenario: see the incredible lessons you learned; the experience you gained; the new understandings you received; and how pleased you are with yourself that you overcame your fears and weren't a prisoner.

Look at all the possible ways you can mitigate the risks to you and still gain most of the benefit: see how you maintained your risk at a level that was acceptable to you so that you still moved forward, and how the mitigations you put in place shifted the benefits of taking action massively in your favor.

Lastly, look at what happens if you decide not to take the risk: look at how you were careful to avoid the trap of not taking the risk as your default answer; how you carefully weighed the opportunities for taking the risk against the potential downsides; how you examined carefully if those downsides could be sufficiently mitigated so that the risk was acceptable to you. But notice that, after seeing the opportunity and risk accurately, you decided consciously and without fear that this wasn't the right choice for you.

See and feel how much clearer it felt to decide what was simply the right answer without fear. Feel how much more ready you are to take the right opportunity (risk) next time.

Keep repeating this three-step process until you see yourself winning all ways.

Let me give you an example of how I used this recently. About a year ago, I got offered an opportunity to invest in something that was very high risk, but very high reward. It was not long after my divorce and so money was still tight.

I knew that there was at least a 50% chance that I would lose my investment, but that if it came off, my returns would be very, very substantial.

So, using the mindset and approach above, I didn't simply say, "It's too risky," "I can't really afford to invest," or "I'll protect what I have." Instead, I looked at the opportunity (notice I said "opportunity" not "risk") and considered the best- and worst-case scenarios.

I saw that in the best case, I would completely financially recover from my divorce and be well set up for the rest of my life. I saw the incredible benefits to me being free to work full-time on my purpose, to be available to my daughters, to be able to give them the best possible life. I saw the incredible knowledge I would gain from being involved in this investment, from the skills and understanding I would gain by taking action now. I saw the people I could network with and get to know. I saw another opportunity to enhance my mindset by putting into practice the thought patterns I have discussed in this chapter.

I saw that in the worst-case scenario, I could well lose all of my investment but that I would still gain all the knowledge, understanding, insights, and connections I mentioned in the best-case scenario. So, I knew I would either win or win big.

While you are doing this, take a look at the most likely scenario as well. As with the best- and worst-case scenarios, find your reward even if you don't get your preferred outcome.

Next, I needed to mitigate the financial risk. Knowing that it was a high-risk investment, I decided the clear and appropriate course of action was only to invest money I was prepared to lose – not money that I wanted to lose or wouldn't care about losing, but an amount that I was OK with losing.

So, I decided upon an amount I was prepared to invest and moved forward. At different times I have financially won and lost on this investment. But overall, I have won massively. I have gained all of the experience, insight, and knowledge I saw was available to me. I have made connections that I never would have accessed otherwise and that will be invaluable to me irrespective of how this investment ultimately turns out.

I have already won.

Can you see how powerful this way of thinking is? Can you start to see the possibilities for your life if you are no longer a prisoner to false fears about risk and can take every opportunity to move forward?

THINGS TO CONSIDER

- Consider: How do you view failure? How do you feel about failing?

- Can you see that failure is part of the natural process of success?

- Can you see the value in simply respecting failure instead of fearing it?

- Consider how the fixed mindset view of failure robs you of all the incredible benefits that failure offers you.

- Consider how past failures have led so many people to their greatest successes. Consider the benefits to you of your past failures.

- Consider whether when "assessing risks" you have really looked at the risks of standing still as well of the risk of taking action. Don't answer straightaway, just consider.

- Can you see how playing it safe is often the biggest risk of all?

CHAPTER 8

HOW TO STOP OVERTHINKING

Overthinking – the art of creating problems that aren't even there.

HOLLY KELLUMS

Overthinking is a disease.

So many people today are *plagued* by their thoughts instead of helped by their thoughts. Their progress is *blocked* by their thinking instead of accelerated. And their problems are *created* by their thinking not solved by them.

And most people have trained their brain not to find answers for them but instead to find evermore problems, risks, and challenges.

Our minds, the very tool we have been given to navigate through life, to set us free, to grow, and to become who we want to be, have instead become the prison, the very thing that keeps most people trapped and stuck, drowning in worries, fears, and options with no structure for working through them.

The incredible problem-solving machine has instead become the amazing problem- creating machine.

Instead of just thinking and processing the thoughts necessary and helpful to us for functioning effectively in our daily lives, we have tipped into **overthinking**, into thinking thoughts that are not simply an unnecessary burden but are actively damaging to us.

Our very thoughts have become toxic.

Most people are no longer simply doing <u>enough thinking</u>, they are doing, way, way, <u>way too much</u>.

This wouldn't be a problem if everyone was overthinking **good thoughts**, but the epidemic is of **negative overthinking**. So the labels don't accurately describe what is happening which makes solving the problem harder.

The world is facing an epidemic of overthinking and all the terrible, awful damage it causes. It's no surprise that mental health issues, stress and anxiety disorders, and cases of depression have skyrocketed over the last 30 years.

ARE YOU IN CONTROL OF YOUR MIND OR IS IT CONTROLLING YOU?

The mind is like water. When it's turbulent, it's difficult to see. When it's calm, everything becomes clear.

– ANONYMOUS

At the root of the overthinking epidemic is that most people have simply lost control of their minds. They don't control their minds; their minds control them.

Most people have, through bad teaching and backwards thinking developed what's called a **ruminating mind**, which is like a washing machine agitating in your head, spinning constantly, day and night. Dr. Robert Glover, the author of *No More Mr. Nice Guy* describes this brilliantly.

A ruminating mind keeps you stuck thinking **about your past**, your perceived mistakes, the opportunities you missed, and replaying your "failures" and the things you got wrong. It shifts your thinking to focus on the bad choices you may have made, on the criticisms and slights you perceive people have made against you, and it uses all of those things to build a case for and constantly remind you of your perceived "defectiveness and inadequacy."

A ruminating mind also blocks your progress by keeping your thinking **about the future** focused on fears, risks, and consequences. It feeds you with a fear of repeating mistakes. It tells you endlessly that you need to gather more information and do more "research" in order to make significant decisions. But this really just keeps you stuck, paralyzed in never-ending analysis.

It convinces you that you can't act until you've considered _every possible outcome of every possible action_, until you've rehearsed every conversation, thought through what you will do (what your script is) for every possible scenario.

In the future, it keeps you focused on the "what ifs?" and constantly feeds you all of the possible negative outcomes of any situation or action. It assumes that there is a perfect way to do everything and that you need to find that "right" answer before you proceed. And even when things are going OK, it shifts your thinking away from what's going well and towards thinking through what's "likely to go wrong next."

Lastly, a ruminating mind keeps you stuck by getting you to endlessly examine and pick through your **perceived inadequacies**. It sets your ego free to compare you to others in ways that make you feel inferior and inadequate, and to measure you by false, arbitrary, and unrealistic standards and expectations. It plays you a constant highlight reel of your mistakes and failures but edits out and/or downplays your successes and achievements.

It gets you to obsess on what people might think about you, how they might react and respond to you. It gets your ego to focus on the validation and approval of others but refuses to believe or accept it when it comes. It causes you to live in fear of rejection and abandonment.

It expects perfection in everything you do and as a result, gives you "imposter syndrome" where it's only a matter of time before you're "found out"; this keeps you fearful of failing and looking foolish.

The combined impact of these thinking patterns is to eat away at your confidence and your ability to create the life you want. They are insidious not only because they fill you with so much doubt, but because as a result, they stop you from acting in your own best interest. _You become paralyzed by your own thoughts_.

This is analysis paralysis.

So, the question about whether you can do something <u>becomes a fact that you didn't</u>, which feeds further doubt. And so, once again, a downward spiral is created.

Ruminating on the past, obsessing about the future, and comparing and measuring yourself <u>always results</u> in a sense of worthlessness, failure, fear, and inadequacy. And through that sense of worthlessness and inadequacy, it keeps you isolated and lonely, because you feel you are not enough for others just as you are. It makes you believe that you have to overcompensate and prove yourself to others in order to be valued, liked, and validated.

But the analysis on which those conclusions are reached, through all that <u>overthinking</u>, isn't accurate. Despite the countless hours of thinking, examining, analyzing, reviewing, scenario planning, data gathering, researching, and so on, the conclusions reached are inaccurate and distorted. That huge effort has led not to greater understanding, but greater **misunderstanding**.

Through overthinking (which as I've already said is really negative thinking disguised as intellectual analysis), all that's created are reinforced distortions, misperceptions, and beliefs about who you are and what you can achieve.

Your mind has tricked you into finding partial, incomplete, and at times plain false "evidence" to support the negative (distorted) beliefs while ignoring information (evidence) that might contradict them.

This is called *confirmation bias*.

What that means is that once you've reached a judgement or decision about something (in this case your value, how you measure up, how well things will go, etc.), your mind, unless you slow down and get in control of your thinking, will look to interpret new evidence as <u>confirmation of your existing beliefs</u>.

It will filter out evidence that goes against them. All "accepted" evidence simply confirms your false sense of inadequacy and failure.

You've actually been on a negative propaganda campaign against yourself that has been disguised as a "fact-finding mission." Like all propaganda, it isn't true and never was.

Remember what Andy taught me: judgement is weakness, observation is power.

In this case, by judging yourself negatively you've programmed your subconscious mind to gather "evidence" to support that false, negative judgement. You've given it a powerful filter that says "even if you find evidence that says I'm great, powerful, incredible, you should ignore this, downplay it, or simply dismiss it."

NO MIND - A REMINDER

As I repeat throughout this book, the foundational skill to becoming who you want to be and creating the life you want to live is gaining control of your mind. It's having the ability to choose one thought over another, to keep the thoughts that help you and make you strong and discard the rest.

So, can you hold 15 seconds of positive thought right now?

If you can, great. If not, consider why you haven't listened to what I said earlier in the book when I told you that this is <u>the foundational skill</u> that you need to master in order to get all the results you want.

You see, I really did mean it.

When Andy first taught me this, I ignored it for years, despite him telling me that it was the most important thing he would ever teach me. I wasted years of my life as a result.

You can now choose to make the same mistake or draw on the benefits of my failure and save yourself that wasted time.

Only you can make the choice to learn the foundational skill to get everything you want in life.

INTELLECTUALIZING OUR EMOTIONS

There is a fundamental misunderstanding that lies at the heart of why so many people suffer with overthinking. And unfortunately, that same misunderstanding is so widespread that the mainstream approaches for dealing with the problem in fact only reinforce it.

So many of the approaches to treat overthinking involve yet more analysis and thinking – the backwards thinking that more of the symptom will be the cure.

And what does that result in? Simply evermore thinking, evermore time in your head, evermore time ruminating, and evermore time stuck in a downward spiral of overthinking and exhaustion.

But what if this is wrong?

What if the problem is not how you think about things but how you *feel* about things?

So often when people are faced with a difficult or uncomfortable situation, they assume that the "difficulty" must be because they lack the **proper knowledge** to do it, not simply that it is **emotionally difficult** for them.

By going into their thoughts instead of their feelings, they are protecting themselves from feeling hurt or upset. They retreat into their minds to avoid the painful emotions they would otherwise feel if they confronted the real challenge.

But because it's not the situation or challenge itself that is the issue but rather how they feel about it, no amount of analysis or thinking will solve it. All the data and analysis doesn't make you feel any better and doesn't give you any answers that work – because you're looking in the wrong place.

Mark Manson describes this brilliantly:

"Intellectualizing situations often distracts us from the difficult truths: that someone flaked on you because they simply don't like you enough to make time for you; that there's no guarantee that your new business will make money; that no matter what you say to someone when you meet them, there's always chance they will reject you; that no matter how much you plan every minute of your vacation, you will not enjoy parts of it; that breaking up with your girlfriend/boyfriend will be incredibly painful no matter how you go about it.

"Analysis paralysis allows us to avoid a difficult emotional situation while feeling like we're accomplishing something by analyzing it. Our minds lead us into an illusion of progress and effort without actual real progress or effort."

Can you see here how the challenge isn't about whether you know what to do <u>but how you feel about the outcome</u>? Can you see that no amount of thinking and analyzing will fundamentally shift the underlying emotional truths?

All the time you spend analyzing and thinking about the "games" the other person is playing by not texting you, you are avoiding the difficult emotional truth that they just don't like you enough to not play games.

But you maintain the fantasy that they do secretly like you; that they just have an issue that they need to deal with because that fantasy protects you from emotional pain. And that avoidance of the truth is why the answers don't really work in reality.

Let me give you an example of how overthinking can work against you, how it keeps you looking at the wrong things and can seriously undermine your progress and confidence.

One of the ways I made a lot of money in the past was through property investing. But before I made any money, I spent a huge amount of wasted time and effort stuck in analysis, blocked in intellectualizing, and sabotaged by overthinking.

I had long seen investing in property as a great way to significantly accelerate my wealth and to create the life that I wanted to live.

So having looked at my options and deciding that property investing was the way to go, I set about reading property books. Pretty quickly I knew everything I really needed to know to get started. **But I didn't**.

Instead, I found and read more books. Each time I looked at a new aspect of property investing, I researched and analyzed it. Sometimes it was about financing a property purchase; sometimes it was about managing the rentals; sometimes it was about dealing with estate agents; sometimes it was learning about which areas were best to buy in and which types of property were the best to buy.

Then it was about the best system for buying property. Should I find investors or just go to the banks? How could I raise money? Should I buy commercial property or residential? Should I build a whole business around this and set up a property investment fund?

Then it was about whether I should buy them personally or set up a company to buy them instead. Then it was about the systems I would need to put in place to manage all the property I was going to buy. Then it was about whether the housing market had peaked and if I had "missed" the opportunity. Then it was about researching the economy and the long-term trends to see if now was a good time to buy or whether I should wait.

The list went on and on. My brain was buzzing. I couldn't switch it off. I felt overwhelmed with all the things I had to do just to get started. I didn't know where to start. At night when I was trying to sleep my mind felt like it was on fire. Thoughts churned over and over in my head as I analyzed every possible scenario, looked at every angle, went through all the risks. I wondered what I would do if interest rates went up: Would I lose my home? Would I go bankrupt? What did it even mean to go bankrupt?

I talked to estate agents endlessly about all my big plans, and to this day I am very grateful for how much they listened to me. I visited and viewed lots of properties as "research." I agonized over the deals I had missed out on and the money I could have made but didn't, because I hadn't completed my preparation and research.

More questions all to be added to the list of work and thoughts and endless analysis I "needed" to do.

I had created problems that weren't even there.

After about 18 months of this, I was exhausted. I was mentally wrung out. I couldn't switch my brain off at all. And I was going around and around in a never-ending loop of questions that only seemed to lead to more questions. I managed to turn answers into questions, into variations, options, and choices – each to be thought over.

And I hadn't even come close to buying one property.

I pretty much decided that it was all too complicated and that I should just forget about it. But even that decision caused me to overthink. I had told so many people about my dream of investing in property. What would they think of me now? Had I failed? What would I say to them when they asked about how it was going?

I had completely lost control of my mind. My mind wasn't working for me to help me buy property. It was sabotaging my efforts to progress. It was finding problems and questions instead of solutions to give me the illusion of progress when in fact I hadn't really moved forward at all. It kept giving me more and more research to do, more and more things to learn, more and more work to "get ready" to act. <u>But without ever acting</u>.

I broke this cycle when I went for lunch with my mentor Andy Shaw. I talked him through where I was at and what I had been doing and the latest deal I was agonizing over. He gave me one simple piece of advice that changed the course of my life.

He smiled at me and simply said, *"Just buy the fucking thing. No matter how it turns out, you'll learn so much from just getting on with it."*

That one simple sentence broke the cycle of rumination, of overthinking, of needing an answer to every question. It made me see that my thinking had become the problem, not the solution.

It made me realize that the problem wasn't my thinking, it was my feelings. I didn't need to <u>know more</u>: I needed to <u>think less</u> and allow space to process my feelings; I needed to let go of my fear of "getting it wrong." But I had been so busy thinking, my feelings never even got a look in.

I didn't need to understand every detail about everything. I simply needed to <u>relax into the uncertainty</u> and get started on the journey.

All my analysis and thinking hadn't led to the root cause because my ego was sabotaging my efforts to progress. It wanted me to stay stuck and it was succeeding.

As Stephen had once told me: Changing wasn't the problem. Not feeling safe to change was.

I drove home from my meeting with Andy and immediately went out and put an offer in on a property. It took me a couple of goes to get it right, but I landed my first deal. Some things went smoothly, some things didn't, but I had made progress. Actual, real tangible progress.

Within two years I became a millionaire.

THE MYTH OF CERTAINTY AND THE "RIGHT" ANSWER

I think the line between analysis and over analysis is where more thinking makes action less likely rather than more likely.

– MARK MANSON

One of my all-time favorite quotes is from Warren Buffet who said, "*I'd rather be approximately right than precisely wrong.*"

What this means is that by getting paralyzed by the fear of making the "wrong decision," many people end up making no decision at all. This means, of course, that they make no progress in life.

Not making a decision is simply making a decision by default. ***To not decide is to decide by accident instead of on purpose.***

Don't get me wrong, you can, on occasion, consciously and deliberately decide to wait and see and to gather more data. That's a perfectly valid thing to do, and something I do frequently. But I do it very deliberately.

That is completely different to simply ducking the decision and being passive.

Most people look for certainty and guarantees before they make any decision, and certainly before any big decision.

The look for the "right answer."

They think that if they wait and gather enough information, they will protect themselves from making a bad decision.

But what if this isn't true, at least in the way that 99% of the world thinks about it? What if that way of thinking has actually blocked you from making numerous decisions that would have been the best ones for you to make (note that I said "best" not "right")?

What if even looking for "right" or "wrong" answers, looking for certainty, isn't even the "right" thing to do? The thing is, the perfectly right answer doesn't exist – certainty is an illusion. There are no guarantees, even if people offer them to you.

No matter what, you will never have the "perfect" information to make a decision. You can never know for sure what will happen and all the possible implications of any decision. And if you did, you could never be 100% certain of making the right decision anyway.

Thinking this way is one of the tricks your ego uses to keep you stuck, playing small, and to block you from making progress.

When you think this way, what you're really telling yourself is that you don't trust that you can handle what might happen; that you don't want to appear to have made a mistake or to have made a bad decision.

This, in turn, means that being indecisive rots away at your confidence.

This is a limiting way of thinking that says you can only progress once you've <u>eliminated risk</u>, have <u>all the information</u>, and have the <u>right answer</u>. But let's examine that thought for a moment, to understand whether it helps you or harms you.

> **SIDE NOTE**
>
> *You should look at all your thoughts this way. Becoming the observer of your thoughts – that is, separating yourself from them so you realize that you aren't your thoughts – is how you change the way you think. Each time you detach and observe your thoughts (not judging, just observing), you give yourself the choice of selecting a different thought if that is better for you.*

Let's take the example of deciding to invest in real estate. You find a potential property to buy, one that looks like it could be a good investment.

You can and should do an appropriate amount of due diligence on the property, the local market, the street the property is on, and the general market conditions. That should take a relatively short period of time (a few hours or days). At the end of that period, you will have enough information to form a reasonable view as to whether to proceed or not.

You will never know for certain if the market is about to crash; you will never be 100% sure that there isn't something wrong with the property; that you will get decent tenants; that interest rates on your loan won't increase; that something else that you don't know about might go wrong.

But if you've done appropriate due diligence, you should know enough to make a well-informed decision. You should know that there's a good chance for you to make a good return on your investment at an acceptable level of risk or not.

But no matter what, a degree of risk will be there. There is always a chance that even after you've done your due diligence, something will go wrong; a black swan event (something major and unforeseen) will occur; or something as simple as a mistake could be made.

But that risk is what makes the opportunity exist.

Do you see this? Risk is the price you pay for opportunity. If there was absolutely no risk, if the returns on your investment were certain, and if it was simple and easy to do, the opportunity wouldn't exist.

Because everyone would be doing it.

And if you wait for perfect information, someone who doesn't need to wait for that perfect information, for that certainty, will execute on the deal quickly and will receive the reward that the risk provides.

This means that by looking for a perfect answer and certainty, you've not only missed the opportunity, but you've only succeeded in creating negative certainty – the certainty of not getting the reward that risk provides.

Through ruminating and overthinking, you can convince yourself that you didn't make a mistake, but is that really true? Is not taking that opportunity really the right answer? And when you're looking for certainty and a "right" answer, can you ever really be in a position to take a risk?

And even if it went "wrong," would that have been a mistake? With everything you learned, with the real-life lessons you have gained, is it really a mistake?

Test your assumptions here. Is it always true that even if something goes wrong, you must have made a mistake? Slow down and consider this.

Things go "wrong" for the 1% all the time, but they don't equate that outcome with them "failing." They don't even think about it that way. They look for the lessons they can take to make them stronger, better, and wiser. They recognize that some of the time their actions, some of their investments, will go wrong.

They realize that, overall, they will make far greater, far faster progress by accepting and embracing risk, by relaxing into the uncertainty of life rather than fearing and avoiding it.

They know they might lose out on specific decisions but that, overall, their lives are much richer for embracing "getting it wrong" sometimes. They don't personalize what happens. They don't see it as being about their value or capabilities. It is simply something that happens – a part of their journey.

But most people do take mistakes very personally; they do think they reflect and reveal their value and capability; they do replay them over and over again in their minds. They convince themselves that their self-worth, their identity, depends on always getting it "right."

And this is what makes the mistakes so painful and the search for certainty and the "right answer" so overwhelming: they are seeking to avoid experiencing that pain of feeling flawed or inadequate again. The risk is no longer just the risk itself but the deep personal wounds associated with the experience of it "going wrong."

They perceive a mistake and replay it. They convince themselves that they are fundamentally flawed and that they must do everything in their power never to make those mistakes again.

But here's the real kicker: your ego, which convinces you that your self-worth depends on you getting it right every time, will criticize and beat you up for having those thoughts; for not being a risk-taker; for not being part of the 1%. Your ego will want you to feel that not being part of the 1% is somehow <u>wrong</u> and reveals a flaw within you.

So, you're damned if you do and damned if you don't. With that thought process, you literally don't allow yourself to win.

Let's take a different example. You see some hot girl or guy you'd like to talk to. Instantly, your ego starts telling you that if you approach them you might get rejected, look like a loser, or be embarrassed or humiliated in some way.

But at the same time, your ego tells you that if you don't approach them, then you're weak, that you're still a loser, that you'll miss the chance, and that someone else will swoop in.

And if they do reject you, your ego beats the crap out of you for "making the mistake" of approaching them and for being such a loser that they did reject you. So, your ego doubles down on both your need to be right and have certainty, and then gets the bonus of beating you up for being rejected and not "being worthy."

But if you never approached them in the first place and heeded your ego's warnings, then of course absolutely nothing happened, which your ego uses as evidence for the "fact" that you just aren't worthy, attractive, good enough, etc.

Then, every night before you go to sleep, your mind imagines all the ways in which they could have been the perfect person for you if only you were braver, better, more confident, etc.

BAD EDUCATION AND THE "RIGHT ANSWER"

One the biggest flaws in how most people are educated is that it teaches the notion that there is always a right answer, and that if you can figure out this right answer, you will get good marks, be rewarded, get a good job, and lead a good life.

Yes, there are clearly certain things that are factual and indisputable. I'm not suggesting that there is never a right answer; some things like math are either right or wrong.

But most of life isn't binary; it's rarely about getting a green tick or a red cross. Most of life is about dealing with people, situations, and goals. It's about creating a life that makes sense to you.

As children, most of us had some strict teachers and some more relaxed teachers; some teachers who loved teaching and were more invested in our growth, and some who didn't like it and just wanted to get through the day; some whose teaching style aligned with our learning style, and some whose teaching style simply didn't work for us. But regardless of these differences, they all laid down a set of rules about how you should behave and what you should think.

Each teacher had a different version of what was right and what wasn't. When you figured out what was right for them, you generally had an easier life. But they all taught you that there was a right answer, and that you got rewarded or not, punished or not, depending on how well you adapted to finding that right answer.

And so, you got taught that this was how you succeed in life, because it was how you succeeded in school.

The only problem is that life doesn't work that way. There is no one to mark your homework after you've done something. And you are the only person in charge of the grading system, because it's about creating a life that makes sense to you.

Imagine if the education system taught students that in life there are actually very few "right" answers; that most of the time, there are simply a set of answers and outcomes, each of which come with a set of possible risks and benefits; that there are no guarantees with any of the choices; that they simply represented a range of possible outcomes.

Imagine if you were taught that risk was simply a fact of life; that sometimes things will go wrong and go against you, even if you do everything "right"; and that, equally, sometimes people get rewarded despite getting lots of things "wrong."

Imagine how differently most people would view the world.

They would see that all choices carry risks and rewards, and so fearing risk was pointless, a complete waste of time, because it was unavoidable.

They would know (and I mean really know) that something going wrong was only a reflection of the fact that something went wrong. It wasn't a measure of whether they were good enough or not. Yes, there were lessons to be learned but that could be done without pain or anguish because it was now simply a process, not something that your self-worth depended on.

They would have the freedom to explore all of their choices, without unconsciously only looking for the unicorn right answer. They would slow down and consider what the right answer for them was, what risks felt right for them to take and which didn't, given their own journey through life.

The search for the right answer is a prison sentence. It's a search that will always remain unfulfilled. It will keep you endlessly searching for more data, when what you need is more clarity around what matters to you, what works for you, and what makes sense to you.

PROCRASTINATION

We are so scared of being judged that we look for every excuse to procrastinate.

– ERICA JONG

When your ego gets you to ruminate and obsess in this way, it gets you to spin your wheels, to work harder and harder without you actually getting anywhere. It gives you the illusion of progress.

One of the biggest tricks it uses to do this is to get you to procrastinate, to put off for "one day" or the "right time" what would most benefit you if done today.

Waiting for the "right time" is a fool's game. And just by playing the game, you lose by default. Your ego convinces you that you are being "smart" by waiting, that you're simply being patient and waiting for the perfect time to act. Most people are astonishing experts at creating bullshit excuses and reasons to delay and ultimately stagnate on any opportunity.

They wait until "one day" to follow their dreams, a day that never quite comes; until one day it's finally too late; until there are no more days, no more chances; until they have wasted that most precious gift of their time, the one resource you can never get back.

Your ego loves "one day" because it gives you the pay-off of not transparently deciding to give up on your dreams while being able to make the choice of false comfort right now.

It's the nearly perfect trap for keeping you stuck, because it's a lie most people want to believe.

The accurate statement would be, **"I'll sacrifice my chance to create the life of my dreams and become the person that I dream of being so that I can wait for the perfect time to start and in the meantime, I will watch TV, play on my phone, watch YouTube etc."**

That's a bit more difficult to swallow but it's also more often the truth.

So I'm clear, there are times when timing matters and judicious and well-considered patience is absolutely the right thing to do. Mindlessly rushing off to do something is almost always counterproductive. Appropriate, intelligent patience is a good thing.

But most people want to believe they are doing this when in fact they are simply avoiding action, even when the opportunity presents itself.

Imagine, instead, if they focused on just doing the next step to get closer to their dreams.

How different would their lives look? How different would your life look if you did the same?

Imagine what your life would look like if for the next month, you *only* focused on taking the next step instead of on excuses and reasons not to progress. Now imagine if you did that for a year, three years, five years, the rest of your life.

But most people don't do this because they look to protect their dreams by never exposing them to reality. They believe that if they have never really tried, then they haven't really failed.

They would rather protect the fantasy that their dreams could happen than expose themselves to the possibility that they might not, despite the fact that this very choice pretty much guarantees that they will never experience their dreams.

The 1% know the difference between good waiting and procrastination. They simply progress when the time is right, but their core tendency is to act, not to wait. They value themselves and their time too much to waste it.

They value their time more than they are concerned about failure. They respect failure instead of fearing it. And so, they don't get into the cycle of overthinking their options.

And that decision is extraordinarily powerful in the journey to them becoming who they want to be and living the life they want to live. It means they can reap the benefits of appropriate patience without the costs of procrastination. It means they calmly consider the right time to execute without the burden of agonizing over that choice. And when they do execute, they can go all in and so maximize their chances of success.

The 1% know this instinctively. And you can relearn it any time you choose.

Imagine what your life would look like if you never procrastinated again, but instead, simply executed when the time was right. You took the risk of things going well, instead of simply focusing on the fear of making the wrong choice.

You would have gone for every good opportunity. Sure, some would have worked and some would have been failures to learn from. But if you really stop and consider it, do you think your life would have been better, richer, more vibrant by simply taking the chance, no matter the outcome? By not agonizing over the choice?

Each time you duck the bold choice your life gets smaller. Each time you go for it your possibilities expand.

All of those combined choices define whether or not your life becomes what you want it to be. By taking the chance, you are saying yes to life and breaking the cycle of overthinking.

Life gives you opportunities or lessons.

So, relax into the uncertainty and embrace the adventures that life offers you.

And start saying "Fuck yes!" to your life right now.

OVERWHELM & FALSE BUSY-NESS

Being busy is not the same as being productive. In fact, being busy is a form of laziness – lazy thinking and indiscriminate action.

– TIM FERRISS

The last area of overthinking that I want to cover is overwhelm. It is another symptom of this disease of overthinking.

Many people are so overwhelmed with everything all of the time that they get nothing done. They feel that no matter what they do, no matter how hard they work, no matter how much effort they put in, they cannot escape from feeling overwhelmed.

And as the means by which we communicate and share information has expanded, our sense of overwhelm has increased. The number of people you would interact with 150 years ago would be relatively small, limited to your family, some people local to you, and occasional letters.

Now we interact with hundreds and often thousands of people each and every day. We have so many channels by which people can contact us – email, text, social media, phone call, video calls, chat rooms. And these go alongside 24-hour global news that bring non-stop news from every corner of the globe, available 24/7/365.

And most people now carry with them the means to interrupt them constantly: their phones. This means every time something happens, no matter how trivial or unimportant, there is a direct and simple means to interrupt you.

This means all of your family can interrupt you whenever they choose; this means all your friends can interrupt you whenever they choose; this means people you work with have the capability to interrupt you <u>whenever they choose</u>.

And on top of that, there are countless apps that most people allow to buzz, ring, and vibrate each time someone posts the latest video of a cat wearing a Darth Vader helmet on social media. And like Pavlov's dog, 99% of people stop whatever they are doing to look at their phones each and every time one of these things happens.

This isn't important information; this is the most useless, pointless, inane bullshit imaginable and yet most people allow this to dominate their lives. They react without thought every time their phone goes off.

I have seen people (and I really wish I was kidding here) answer their phones in public toilets. Men standing at urinals frantically reaching for their phones while they're taking a leak.

I have heard (again I really wish I was kidding) people taking a dump and still answering their phones and having conversations at the same time!

In all seriousness, take a moment to consider the breathtaking insanity of this – an insanity that most people do to themselves.

If you are in the bathroom, do you really need to answer the phone, check your messages, update your social media?

Tai Lopez recently posted research findings that showed that the average human's attention span has dropped to around eight seconds, whereas the average goldfish's is around 12 seconds. So yes, the average human has less ability to concentrate than a fucking goldfish!

Ask yourself these simple questions: How many of these interruptions are necessary? How many of them require immediate attention? How many of them help get work done?

How many of these interruptions required people to interrupt their time going to the bathroom? I would guess pretty much zero. Maybe one in a thousand, which is still essentially zero.

Most people have become incredibly busy doing nothing! We are overwhelmed with the meaningless, the pointless, and the valueless. We become preoccupied with the latest nonsense on social media and then with people's comments and reactions to the nonsense.

We get taken in with the manufactured drama and false urgency of the 24-hour news and then with people's reactions to the manufactured and false drama, including a general kind of manufactured outrage, which starts the cycle all over.

We have filled up our lives with meaningless, valueless, junk food information and interactions, and then wonder why we feel overwhelmed. We allow ourselves to be interrupted every few seconds, and then wonder why our ability to concentrate is decimated and we can't get things done.

And so most people are going nowhere fast. Their lives are filled with unfocused busyness, expending time, money, and effort in multiple different directions.

The net result? Not very much.

The next time you are around people, listen to how frequently and without thought they speak of how busy they are, almost as a badge of honor. Notice that they don't talk about how **productive** they are, or how much they've achieved, simply how much they **have to do**.

It is almost a means of representing their value, like the busyness itself gives them worth.

Very few realize (by which I mean, live as a way of life) that if work isn't clearly and tightly focused towards a well-understood goal, it is largely worthless.

Only when you become conscious of this collective insanity can you become free of it. But the first step is to realize that you are creating the problem. It is not a problem that exists outside of you; it is a problem that you have allowed to develop within you by the absence of conscious thought and consideration.

So, the good and bad news is that you have created the problem and so you can un-create it.

The path to being free from overwhelm is to become conscious of it and put in place structures and routines for your thoughts and actions that don't simply manage overwhelm but actually prevent it from building up in the first place.

THE POWER OF SAYING "NO"

The difference between successful people and very successful people is that very successful people say "no" to almost everything.

– WARREN BUFFETT

So much of overwhelm comes from not simply saying "No" to things that don't have any benefit for you, don't advance your purpose, plans, and agenda, and fill up your life with meaningless crap.

The problem is that the low value and meaningless crowds out the time and mental space that you could otherwise direct towards becoming who you want to be and creating the life you want to live.

Think of your day as a container, with a fixed amount space and capacity. Every day you get to choose what goes into that container: how much good stuff, how much negative stuff, how much that helps you, and how much that works against you.

Imagine if you could see each day (container) from your life so far. If you looked at the thousands of containers that made up your life so far, how many of them contain more negative, meaningless, and unhelpful stuff than you would like? Can you see how this creates the picture, the reality of your life?

Now imagine if you predominantly filled each container <u>for the rest of your life</u> with good stuff. Can you see how that would change the picture?

But to make space for the good stuff – the thoughts, choices, actions, experiences, and feelings that help you – you need to start saying "No" to everything else.

This might sound painful and like hard work but that's your ego playing tricks on you. We're talking about creating the life you dream of, the life that will bring you complete freedom, joy, success on your terms, all the experiences you desire, all the feelings about yourself that you would love to have.

And it simply requires making space for it. It means removing the weeds in your mind so that there's only room for flowers.

HOW TO GET FREE FROM OVERWHELM

There are some really simple day-to-day things that you can do that will make an immediate difference to your sense of overwhelm. They involve simple daily practices that, if applied, will dissolve so much of the overwhelm that so many suffer from.

As you go through this, watch your ego immediately throw up all kinds of reasons, rationalizations, arguments, and justifications for why what I'm saying "isn't realistic" – that it's too hard, that you can't do it because [insert excuse here]. Don't judge it or resist it when it happens, just slow down and observe your thoughts. Recognize that creating your dream life and joining the 1% who create life on their terms means not doing what the 99% do.

I can't make you do this. I know the incredible benefits to your life; the riches you can create; the success you have in your grasp; the natural, effortless confidence that you can unleash if you take these steps. But ultimately, only you can choose to do it.

First of all, TURN OFF YOUR PHONE! In the world today, you cannot avoid some sense of overwhelm if you are slave to your phone. So, **TURN IT OFF**.

Decide consciously and deliberately when to turn it on, when to allow yourself to be contacted. That leaves the rest of your time to be able to be productive. If you have to leave your phone on for whatever reason, make sure you have nearly all the notifications turned off.

The only notifications on my phone that I have switched on are for a small and carefully selected group of people for texts and calls. That's it. Everything else is switched off.

When I first did this, I simply couldn't believe the change it made to my productivity and feelings of overwhelm. I was staggered at the progress I was able to make.

I went from having 50 or 60 or sometimes more than 100 notifications a day to one or two. It felt strange, even uncomfortable at first, but when I spent some time considering the benefits and costs of the countless interruptions, it became a pretty straightforward choice.

When I first did this, I'll admit that I found it hard – very hard.

Previously, I was unquestionably, completely addicted to my phone. But something interesting happened. After a few days, I noticed how much less distracted I was; how much more present I was; how much easier it was to focus to get done the things I needed; how many great ideas I started having. I had freed my mind from *being a slave to my phone*.

If you want to massively expand your capacity to transform your life, give yourself the gift of trying this for a few days. You will surprise yourself with how little you want to go back to being addicted to your phone.

Next, don't watch the news.

I struggle to put into words the difference this made to my life. If you want to truly see the madness of the 99%, switch off all news for a week. Notice how the world doesn't end for you, life goes on pretty much as it did before, and that day-to-day life is completely OK.

Watch how 99% of people complain, get angry, irritated, frustrated, sad, upset, or feel helpless as a result of a set of things that have happened (and therefore that you can do nothing about).

And even though your day-to-day life really hasn't changed, notice how much less of your time you spend feeling those negative feelings.

Here's the problem: today's 24-hour news cycle requires those networks to find, create, and often manufacture "news" to fill 24 hours of airtime. EVERY. SINGLE. DAY.

And then they need to find ways to get you to watch and engage with it. To do that, they need to create an emotional pull, which is most easily done by manufacturing controversy, by interviewing people who will make provocative and so newsworthy statements, and by creating conflict and arguments.

So much "news" is manufactured drama and fake urgency. That isn't a political statement. This is about how the media organizations seek engagement with you, not about any specific subject or political viewpoint.

So, despite what most people think, you are rarely better informed by watching the news. You are simply exposed to more negativity that makes very little difference to your day-to-day life.

Think back over the last year. Imagine if you had not read a single newspaper, not watched a single news broadcast. How much would your life have been negatively affected?

Now imagine if your mind had been free from all that false drama, fake urgency, manufactured outrage for the last 12 months. Do you think your mind would have been calmer? Do you think you would have had more mental space to think about the things that would have made a massive difference to your life? More mental space to create the life you dream of?

Can you see that by simply looking at the benefits and costs of these previously unconscious decisions, how you start to direct your life in the way you want rather than in the ways others want?

KNOW YOUR PRIORITIES

One of the most important lessons I learned was that I needed to know and live to my priorities, and that not 1 in 100 people know their priorities and could tell you what they were if asked.

It's only by knowing what *is important* that you can know what *isn't*.

And knowing what isn't important is the first step to dropping it and so reducing your overwhelm.

Every day I have four priorities that I focus on; that I care deeply about; that I invest in, focus on, and execute. No matter what. I go all in on these every day.

They are my mindset, my family, my business, and my health.

By knowing that list (yours may be the same or different, but know it), I know that other things are less important, and less worthy of my energy, attention, and focus.

That list is the reference point for what I emotionally invest in and just as importantly **WHAT I DON'T**.

It means that when challenges present themselves, when I'm dealing with life day to day, I can ask myself simply, "Is this one of my priorities?"

Anything that isn't one of those four gets chosen with great care, because by definition, it's time, energy, and focus away from what I know matters most to me.

I may still do it *but it now becomes a conscious choice, not an unconscious one*.

Then all the noise that fills up so many people's lives remains just that: background noise. I'm aware that it's there, but I'm not invested in it or affected by it.

There's a lot of conversation right now about the virtues of "not giving a fuck." But it's not giving a fuck that's the problem. It's giving a fuck about too many unimportant and often irrelevant things that distract you from creating your life on your terms.

Knowing your priorities means you can easily and without effort stop sweating the small stuff.

This matters, because being busy is NOT the same as doing the things that matter.

Ask almost anyone these days how they are and nine times out of ten the answer will be "busy." It is almost as if they're scared of not only not being busy but not being seen to be busy. And so, the world is rushing around being busy and achieving very little of what matters most to them.

You may have heard of the Pareto Principle which says that 80% of your results come from just 20% of your actions. And this is almost always true.

In fact, more recent studies have shown that it's even more skewed so that 90% or 95% of your results come from only 5% or 10% of your actions.

So, it's factually correct to say that creating the life you want rarely requires you rushing around doing lots of things.

It absolutely requires you consistently focusing on the most important things. These are usually the things that seem hard, that scare you, and that take you outside your comfort zone.

Because those feelings are a guide. They light the road to the life you want.

Imagine how different your life would be if you stopped being so busy, eliminated all the noise and distractions, and did only the 5% or 10% of things that really mattered.

Then you could step away from the crazy herd mentality that being busy is good, and step into the life you really want.

JUST TAKE THE NEXT STEP

When you are creating the life you desire, don't focus on all the things you have to do to create it.

That takes something you love (your dream life) and turns it into hard work, which is pretty much the fastest way to destroy your progress.

Instead, still your mind, accept that everything that needs to get done will get done at the right time in the right way – maybe not to the deadlines you originally thought or that others expect, but everything will get done when the time is right.

How do I know this? Well, despite all the feelings of overwhelm in the past, you're still here, you've made it to today, so everything necessary for that to happen has happened.

Next, allow yourself to daydream. Allow yourself to see your dream life as already done, already created. Enjoy the feeling of it being done.

Then focus on the next step you have to take to create that life and **only** on that step. Don't try to start five other things or look at five other options.

Do whatever you need to do to complete it. Go about it in a workmanlike way until it is done.

Then rinse and repeat.

Imagine if you did this for one year, three years, five years, or even the rest of your life.

Instead of feeling overwhelmed with bad feelings, you would create amazing feelings and continual progress.

Just imagine how quickly you could create the life of your dreams then.

The 1% who become who they want to be and create the life they want to live, don't spend time dwelling on the past or fearing the future. They simply take the next step.

They do whatever they need to do to get to the next step, and then the next and then the next.

They learn the lessons they need to learn along the way. They overcome the obstacles placed before them, grateful that the challenges and "failures" are making them stronger, wiser, and better prepared to create what they desire.

They take calm, focused, consistent daily action.

Your ego loves you talking about what you could have done once the opportunity has passed. It's a great way to keep you feeling stuck and playing small.

Today, just decide to take the next step; that's all, nothing more. Do the same tomorrow and then the next day.

And sooner than you can imagine, your world will transform.

THINGS TO CONSIDER

- Do you now control your mind or does your mind still control you?

- Have you yet been able to hold the 15 seconds of positive thought and bring in No Mind? Have you attempted this yet? If not, consider if you still think there is anything more important for you to do.

- Are you able to do only the thinking required to deal with any situation or circumstance, or do you overthink? Consider if you want to continue overthinking anymore.

- Do you use intellectual analysis to distract you from facing uncomfortable emotional truths?

- Consider the situations or challenges you are facing right now. Do you need more information and analysis in order to progress or do you simply need to feel safe to do so?

- Is your analysis making progress more likely or less?

- Consider that risk is necessary for opportunity to exist. If there was no risk and it was easy, then everybody would be doing it – in which case, there would be no opportunity.

- Consider: Have you fallen for the myth of the "right answer"?

- Can you see that being busy is not the same as being productive? And that uncontrolled busyness is actually a form of laziness?

CHAPTER 9

HOW TO ELIMINATE
FEAR, WORRY & DOUBT

Worry pretends to be necessary but serves no useful purpose.

ECKHART TOLLE

Would you like to never worry again?

I get that this probably sounds like nothing more than a fantasy. The kind of thing where your ego says, "Of course I wish I never worried again, but don't be so stupid. That will never happen."

I understand that reaction and it was one I had myself until I was shown "the way" on this by Andy and Stephen. They showed me the path to never needing to worry, fear, or doubt again; the path to living carefree no matter what.

So just for a few moments, tell your ego to give you a break and allow you a few minutes to imagine this: imagine what your life would look and feel like without any fear, worry, or doubt.

Can you imagine for a moment what your life would be like if you completely eliminated worry from your life?

Can you imagine how much you would be able to achieve, how much success you would create, how much fun and enjoyment you would have, and how light and easy your journey through life would feel?

Can you imagine how much better your life would be, if instead of worrying, you could just get on and simply deal with any situations that you needed to?

Can you imagine how incredible your progress would be if all of your time and energy was freed up to create, to make progress, and to do what you love instead of being wasted on anxiety and worries?

Instead of, say, 30% of your time and energy being used to propel you forward, imagine that 70%, 80%, or even 100% was directed towards creating the life you want.

Well, despite what your ego may be telling you, this is not only entirely possible, it is your natural state. Worrying was a bad habit that you learned to do. You learned this from the bad habits of your parents, teachers, friends, and broader society.

To be clear, I am not judging anyone for worrying. I have done plenty myself. And I lost a huge amount of my life to worrying about a whole heap of things that never happened. This is time that I will never get back.

So, I am simply telling you that this is a bad habit that works against you; that worrying is a complete and total waste of time; that like all bad habits, it can be changed with clear, accurate thinking.

And I'll show you how.

THE VICIOUS CYCLE OF WORRYING

Right now, there is an anxiety epidemic. The number of people suffering from anxiety has exploded in recent years, despite that, by any historical measure, we actually live in one of the safest times in human history.

Worry, fear, and anxiety have become a default state for so many. It has become a reflex reaction to almost anything that happens – or even when nothing happens at all. And when they can't find something, when their non-specific anxiety needs something to land on, they simply pick something so at least the anxiety has an outlet, a "reason," a "cause."

Here's how this works.

At some point in your childhood, you saw someone, most likely someone who was looking after you, be fearful, scared, or anxious about something. Because you didn't yet fully understand the world, you likely assumed you were in some kind of danger.

And because children model what their parents and teachers do, not what they say to do, you will have started to pick up this bad habit.

So, you started to learn (get programmed) that "this is what we do."

Without structured, accurate thinking being given to you, without enough explanation or understanding about what was happening, you began to learn that this was the appropriate response to situations. It became what you learned that you "should" do. And remember that anything you "should" do is something that you were programmed to do. "Shoulds" are learned patterns of behavior, not natural patterns of behavior.

Again, I want to be clear: I am not judging anyone (your parents, my parents, your teachers, or my teachers) in any way about this. I want you to see how you learned to worry, so you can effectively unlearn it.

You got taught that this was a "normal" reaction to situations and circumstances: to worry, be fearful, or anxious; to examine and explore, often in great and vivid detail, all the possible ways things could go "wrong" or turn out "badly"; to focus your mind's incredible imaginative, creative, and analytical power on the ways things could turn out badly; to fill your mind with these thoughts.

To be clear, this isn't what definitely will happen, just what could, possibly, or may happen.

Your ego, like those of your parents and teachers before them, did one of its core tricks: to take something seemingly good and turn it into a weapon to be used against you.

Your ego told you that by scanning the horizon for all the scary things that could happen to you that you were keeping yourself "safe," and that therefore you were putting yourself in danger if you didn't. It wasn't enough to simply be aware of risks or genuine dangers. You needed to be on high alert about them, because if you let your guard down (by relaxing and not worrying) you were putting yourself at risk.

This meant that you ended up feeling anxious whenever you caught yourself not feeling anxious – at which point it became a default state.

Over time, your ego then persuaded you that it is responsible to worry. It was not simply something a lot of people might do; it was not just a response to a clear and present danger. It was your responsibility to worry; that you were somehow irresponsible if you didn't. And so, it then became locked in behavior.

Can you see the tricks, the breadcrumb trail, your ego is laying for you here? It's leading you right into a trap, a prison that very few ever escape from.

This is why so many people worry or get anxious about lots of little things; about being late for an appointment; about missing their train; about whether they said the wrong thing and accidently upset someone; about whether the night out they are organizing will go well; about whether the work they did yesterday was good enough; about whether they ate too much food or too little, drunk too much coffee and not enough water; about whether the meeting they have tomorrow will go well or badly.

Because it is default behavior – "responsible" behavior – to worry.

At the same time, all these small worries are mixed in with all kinds of big worries; is there something wrong with my health; will I have enough money to pay my bills; will I lose my job; will I spend my life alone; am I a good parent/friend/partner/sibling/person; will I get attacked; will I ever live the life that I want; am I good-looking/charming/talented enough?

Soon enough they create a huge mental library of things that they can, do, and will worry about. They have literally focused their minds on creating, managing, and storing an ever-increasing catalogue of reasons to worry.

Do you see how this works? Can you see how destructive it is? Can you see why no thought stands still? That every thought helps you or harms you? Can you see how allowing these chaotic worry thoughts to take up space in your mind causes you evermore pain and problems? It isn't neutral; it is actively damaging.

Can you see how worry and fear are like a cancer that simply grows inside your mind, crushing out all the good thoughts and replacing them with bad ones – until eventually there is nothing left apart from bad thoughts?

Don't feel bad if this is you too. Be delighted that you can start to see the insanity that keeps most of the world a prisoner for nearly their whole lives. Be delighted with yourself for having uncovered the problem and for finding the material that will show you how to break this habit for good.

THE TRUE 'WORRY PRICE'

***Of all the liars in the world, some of the worst are
your own fears.***

– RUDYARD KIPLING

Have you ever looked at what worry really means? I had never looked at the dictionary definition of worry until my friend Andy Shaw mentioned it in one of his courses.

But looking it up for myself and spending some time thinking about it made me see the insanity of worry. I spent quite some time just considering this definition after reading it for the first time and wondering why I had given over any of my time to worrying.

The *Cambridge English Dictionary* defines worry as:

"To make someone feel unhappy and frightened because of problems or unpleasant things that might happen."

Worry is by definition an act of making yourself feel unhappy and frightened because of things that *might* happen: not have happened; not are happening; not definitely will happen; but simply might happen.

Worry is the act of causing yourself pain, unhappiness, and fear over a possibility. It is experiencing a scenario that you've decided will cause you pain and problems without those problems ever actually needing to exist. It is not the act of solving your problems, making them better, or doing anything productive. It is the opposite. It is experiencing the pain without the cause actually being there.

It is by definition an act of self-abuse and self-harm. And if you choose to continue to worry, then you are choosing to be abusive towards yourself. Again, don't let your ego use this to make you feel bad. Just observe your feelings here. Do not judge. As you observe the fact that you have been self-harming and that worrying serves no purpose, you can start to let it go.

You like 99% of people didn't know you were self-harming, so give yourself a free pass on this. You are now conscious of the choice though. This means, maybe for the first time, you have the ability to make a different choice.

So, before I show you how to cure worry, fear, and anxiety, I want you to understand what the costs of the habit of worrying are – and the incredible, astonishing benefits awaiting you when you give up the need to worry.

We've already seen that on its own, worry is an act of self-harm that takes away your day-to-day peace and happiness. But the true costs are actually far deeper.

SWITCHING OFF YOUR INCREDIBLE
PROBLEM-SOLVING MACHINE

One of the biggest costs of fear, worry, and anxiety is that far from keeping you safe, it actually blocks you from solving the very problem, issue, or challenge that is causing you to worry in the first place. Our ego's like to convince us that worrying helps you to prepare, when in fact the exact opposite is true.

Not only do worry and fear block you from seeing the solutions that are right in front of you, they stop you from taking action even when you do.

When your mind is fearful, anxious, or worried, it blocks your ability to think accurately, clearly, or creatively. Your mind becomes so filled with fears and worries that your mental energy gets focused on and dominated by these thoughts, by the consequences of what could go wrong.

Your mind is so busy, so filled up with processing all of these terrible consequences that it goes into fight or flight mode, which is often referred to as your reptilian brain. This next section is based on Dr. Paul McLean's work on the triune brain.

The reptilian brain is the most primitive part of your brain and is brilliant at helping you deal with a number of specific scenarios to react (not respond) to without thought. So, it would help you immediately react without thought if you were about to crash your car; it would help you fight back if you were being attacked. It protects our lives much faster than it would take us to activate our reasoning capabilities to do the same actions.

But as important and necessary as it is, you don't want it controlling your day-to-day thoughts and actions. This part of our brain is *focused on our survival* and so it gets scared very easily and stops us from doing what we want to do rather than simply what helps us to survive.

So when your reptilian brain is in control you won't try new things, you won't get creative, and you won't think clearly. In fact, you'll hardly be thinking at all. You'll be operating on pure instinct.

In this mode, your higher brain functions in the limbic brain. The neocortex can hardly function, yet these parts of your brain are where your ideas, intuition, and creativity come from.

Being fearful or worried means you are switching on the least helpful parts of your brain to solve the problem. To solve a modern-day issue, you are using the parts of your brain that are there to help you fight wild animals. It's the wrong tool for the job!

Can you see now the insanity of thinking that worrying keeps you safe?

The problem is that our reptilian brains do not have the ability to distinguish between life-threatening situations and things that we really don't like but don't actually threaten our survival, like losing your job, divorce, etc. And so, because most people have switched on their reptilian brains through worry, they stay in fight or flight mode (at low or high levels) even when there is no clear and present danger. This means that they can't access the power of their higher brains – the part of their brains that can actually solve the problems or challenges they are facing.

It is sensible, mature, and right to be aware and conscious of the challenges you may face and to take considered action to bring about the outcome you desire or to avoid the outcome you wish to avoid.

But that is not the same as worrying about it. You can undertake all the analysis, planning, and preparation to create your best life. But the outcome, good or bad, will not improve *in any way* by you worrying about it.

There's not a karmic worry price you must pay in order to "buy" a good outcome. That just means you end up worrying about not worrying! All that does is create pain and stops you from having the calm, clear mind that will give you the answers you need to solve whatever problem you face.

GETTING MORE OF WHAT YOU FEAR

If you simply stayed in fight or flight mode (in your reptilian brain) for short periods, that would be one thing. But most people spend nearly their entire lives in some level of fear, worry, or anxiety. They lose, or rather **they sacrifice,** years of their precious lives to this torment.

But here's the bigger problem.

The way our minds work is that we get more of whatever we focus on. Our minds are perceptual machines filtering in and out of our conscious awareness those things that align with our dominant thoughts. So if you see the world through the lens of fear, your mind will faithfully go out and find **by default** all manner of things for you to be scared of and worried about.

And because that is the filter you have set on how you see the world, your mind automatically filters out things that are irrelevant according to that perception. Those irrelevant things may include all the great stuff that is happening and available to you; all the possibilities; all the opportunities that may be right there in front you. But they get filtered out by your mind. And this skews the picture and makes you even more fearful. It doesn't matter whether it's true or accurate. It matters what you perceive to be true and accurate.

Think of it being a little bit like YouTube and the videos it shows you. There are a huge number of videos available on YouTube and it can't show you them all. YouTube looks at the videos you've watched before and then filters the videos it presents to you in line with the preferences you have expressed through what you have watched previously. You may not have gone and deliberately set any preferences at all. YouTube has simply learned this by tracking your behavior.

If you watch lots of videos on cute puppies, YouTube will show you more videos of cute puppies. If someone else watches countless videos of natural disasters, YouTube will show them more videos like that (and not any cute puppies!). Both exist, both are real and true, but one is clearly more likely to make most people feel afraid. YouTube will keep showing more and more of the natural disaster videos until your preferences change.

Your mind operates in exactly the same way.

When you focus on your worries and fears, you end up creating more reasons for those worries and fears to exist. So, because of this stupid, shortsighted, toxic teaching, the vast majority of 99% of people's thoughts are about what they don't want, what they're scared of, and what they don't like and are desperate to avoid.

They are not about finding their purpose, their perfect partner, creating a life of financial freedom, their dream home.

They want their dreams, but all of their thoughts and decisions are subconsciously about managing their fears.

So, they are sabotaging themselves on an industrial scale.

THE POWER OF POSSIBILITY VS CONSEQUENCE

Fear is an idea crippling, experience crushing, success stalling inhibitor inflicted only by yourself.

– STEPHANIE MELISH

One of the biggest differences between the 1% who become who they want to be and create the life they want to live and everyone else is the unconscious framework they have for making decisions about their lives.

This framework shapes how they see the world, how they view, frame, and process the decisions and choices they face day to day. You were born with this same framework, this same way of looking at the world. Everybody was. The only difference is that the 1% never lost this ability and never had it programmed out of them.

The 1% focus on possibilities; the 99% focus on consequences.

This base framework of possibility versus consequence informs so many decisions –from the daily and the mundane to the large and life changing. It determines where our mind's power is focused and so what we create in our lives.

Our focus determines whether we create more possibility and more opportunity, or more consequence and more work to avoid those consequences.

The 1% stay aware of and prepared for whatever may happen, in order to take advantage of the abundance of opportunities they see around them. They are curious and filled with excitement about the possibilities that life offers and so they are focused on growth instead of security.

This doesn't mean they are reckless – beware your ego trying to tell you that you have to give up your security to achieve your success. That kind of binary thinking is a trick your ego loves to use to keep you stuck.

It means looking at the *primary driver* of your decisions and whether it drives you towards your dreams and desires – towards becoming who you want to be – or whether it takes you away from those dreams.

It means taking sensible, worthwhile steps to mitigate your risks and protect your position, and to focus on and move towards your dreams and seizing opportunity as it occurs.

Let me give you an example.

When Elon Musk sold PayPal, he personally made around $200m. As soon as he got the money, he invested $100m to start up Tesla, $90m to start up SpaceX and $10m to start up SolarCity. He is now worth over $20bn as a direct result.

Most people would have happily retired at that point, but Elon Musk was so curious and excited about the possibilities that life held that he couldn't wait to get started. He focused on what he could create, not on what he could lose.

I would only make a minor tweak to his plans if I had faced the same choices. He could have set $10m aside, to mitigate his risks and guarantee a life of luxury no matter what.

But the overall direction is the same.

Let's take a small-scale, day-to-day example.

Let's say you saw the possibility of making money from real estate and that you could raise the money to start investing by refinancing your main home. You recognize that this path offers you the opportunity to create wealth, potentially significant wealth, with all the benefits to your life that brings.

But it also entails a degree of risk.

Does your mind now drift to the opportunity, to the dream of the wealth, or to the fear of loss? Or maybe you get really excited about the idea of the wealth but that excitement is ultimately overtaken and then blocked by the fear of loss.

Take a moment to feel your answer here. Remember, it is in the consideration of these often-hidden thought patterns that you uncover the blocks – the bugs in your thinking that are blocking your natural success mindset.

It is only by observing your thoughts and reactions, by becoming conscious of these bugs that you can change them.

Lots of people love the idea of the wealth that the property investment could bring but get blocked at the idea stage. After the idea stage, their focus would drift to consequence and away from possibility. For the 1%, however, their focus on the possibility would grow.

Over time, this difference in focus would lead to those who did invest in a first property having more wealth that they could reinvest in a second property, and then a third and so on. And the irony of that is that ultimately, they would have <u>much less to be fearful of</u> because they would be independently wealthy and not dependent on a wage for their financial well-being.

So, what's your current default setting? Do you make your decisions based on possibility and opportunity or based on fear and consequence?

When something happens, such as a chance to put yourself in the spotlight, a new job or business opportunity, some hot girl/guy you want to talk to, etc., do you immediately start to consider all the things that could go wrong?

Or do you look for the possibilities that the situation would offer you no matter the outcome?

Two of the most important reasons that people aren't happy with themselves or their lives are: they don't know what they want, and they don't take the opportunities that life presents them anyway.

Then they wonder why things don't "work out for them."

The problem is that their thinking and so their decision-making is almost entirely defined by their fears. The incredible possibilities of what could go right is either hardly considered at all or instantly dismissed.

Their thinking is that they don't expect things to work out for them so they filter out the good that's right in front of them. In a world of opportunity unprecedented in human history, they convince themselves time and again that playing it safe is the "smart call."

And so, the potential for another life withers and dies. Has this been you too, more than you'd like to admit?

Don't beat yourself up if it has. Simply being aware and honest enough with yourself to acknowledge it is the most critical step to changing it. So be delighted with yourself.

Then the next time an opportunity comes up, take a few minutes and allow yourself to consider all the amazing things that could go right. See all the benefits that could flow into your life by meeting your perfect partner, by finding a job that you love, by starting the business you've always dreamed of.

Allow yourself to daydream. Then see how right it feels to throw those possibilities away to just quiet your fears. Then you can start to see the true costs of living a life defined by your fears.

YOUR FEARS ARE YOUR LIMITS

That difference in focus between opportunity and consequence creates another knock-on impact: the limits you create for your life.

These are not the <u>real limits</u> to what you could achieve, the success you could create, the money you could make, or the relationships you could have.

Your fears are the self-created limits you impose on your own life.

Here's how this works.

Each fear you have, each fear that you choose to accept instead of overcoming, sets a limit on your life. It represents something you have chosen not to do; a path you will not walk down; a choice you will not make; a door you will not open; an opportunity you will not take.

The fear sets the boundaries of what you can experience; of how big your dreams can be; how much you can achieve; how good you can feel; the success you can have. Everything.

Every single fear is you choosing, consciously or unconsciously, to close the door on something you could otherwise be, do, or have. It is you shutting doors in your own face.

Let's say you have a fear of getting rejected. This may be a big fear or a low-level fear, but any and every time it stops you, your life becomes less than it could otherwise be.

Imagine you are standing in the queue at a coffee shop, and you see someone who you would love to go and talk to, ask out, maybe go on a date with. You think they're amazing, gorgeous, and incredible. You want to go and talk to them, but the second that desire kicks in, so does your fear that they will turn around and reject you out of hand – "humiliate" you in front of "everyone."

Can you see how you've moved straight to consequence instead of opportunity?

You don't know they will reject you. You have absolutely no idea, because you haven't approached them. You were blocked by your fear.

For all you know they could be just waiting for you to go and speak to them; they could be your perfect partner and life has just presented to them to you; they could be someone you have a really great chat with and enjoy a few minutes talking to; they could be someone for you to learn exactly what you needed to learn to approach your perfect partner when you do meet them.

Maybe, even if they're not interested, they will be kind, respectful, and polite and you've made their day and made them feel great because you approached them and let them know you were interested in them. Maybe that's exactly what they needed to hear because they had been feeling a bit shit about themselves and it made them feel amazing that someone liked them enough to overcome their fear and ask them out.

Maybe, even if they do reject you out of hand and you realize it wasn't that hard to deal with actually, that this lesson, this realization of the truth sets you free to live your life without the fear of rejection that has held you back for so long.

So, you either got the date or you got the lesson. Either way you won or won big.

Every limit you have is in some way, shape, or form, a fear. But fears aren't facts. They are our *perception* of what *might* happen, not what will.

When you know that every fear is a limit, you need to consider very carefully what you will allow yourself to be afraid of.

You stop allowing yourself to be entirely indiscriminate with your fears; you slow down enough to explore the costs of your fears.

The problem with any fear is that it keeps you stuck, because your ego gets you to only look at the risks of taking action. It never gets you to clearly and accurately examine the costs of **not taking action**. The underlying (and entirely false) assumption is that standing still is the safe option.

Which isn't true 99% of the time.

Because every step you take in the direction of the life you want to live and becoming the person you want to be is a victory.

And when you see this truth, when you look at life accurately instead of through the warped and twisted lens of fear, you can see that your fears don't keep you safe at all.

Then (and only then) do you break through your self-imposed limits; only then do you start to see the real and incredible possibilities for your life.

ELIMINATING THE HABIT OF FEAR AND WORRY

Fear is not real. The only place that fear can exist is in our thoughts about the future. It is a product of our imagination causing us to fear things that at present do not exist and may never exist. That is near insanity. Do not misunderstand me, danger is very real but fear is a choice.

– CYPHER RAIGE

The rest of this chapter is going to cover the process of not simply how to rid yourself of worry, but how to rid yourself of *any need to worry*. When it comes to worry, fear, and anxiety, prevention is far more effective than cure.

I don't want to teach you how to manage and cope with these states. I will show you how to remove them, because when you remove them through accurate, structured thinking, you won't need to find ways of managing and coping.

You will simply no longer worry, which will free up all of that effort to focus on creating the life you dream of. When you replace the faulty, unhelpful thinking patterns that cause worry and fear with the structured, helpful ones that return you to your natural, non-worrying ways of thinking, the worry habit just falls away.

DON'T TRUST YOUR FEARS

Always remember: there is <u>the situation that you are facing</u> and there are the fears and worries you have <u>about the situation</u> you are facing.

This misunderstanding lies at the heart of so many fears and worries. And it is in that misunderstanding that fears and worries grow, escalate, and come to overwhelm and dominate the lives of so many people.

One is **what is actually happening**; the second is **the illusion** of what might, could, or possibly happen – and what it might, could, or possibly mean.

Be very aware of that difference and conscious not to mix up the two.

When I was at university, I had a period where I worried intensely about how well I would do in my degree. I had generally done really well in all my grades and was flying high until, for various reasons, I got a few bad marks.

Suddenly my thinking went from how well things <u>were going</u> to how badly things <u>could go</u>. My thoughts, worries, and fears started drifting out further and further into the future. Soon it wasn't simply about how good a degree I would get, to what kind of job could I get, or if I really fucked things up, would I get a job at all?

Was I screwing up the rest of my life, spending a lot of money and taking on significant debts to get nothing of value in the end? Was I wasting three years of my life? Was this something I would look back on and see as some kind of negative turning point in my life? The point where "everything" went wrong for me?

Can you see the difference between the actual situation (a run of bad marks) and my fears about the situation (a bad job, no job, massive debt for nothing, screwing up the rest of my life)?

I caused myself untold pain not from the reality of some bad marks but from the illusions created in my mind about what those bad marks meant. I had stopped seeing the real situation and focused on a whole set of potential consequences that hadn't happened, weren't happening, and may never happen.

Like so many worries, this (screwing up my life) didn't come to pass. I did very well at university. I had entirely wasted my time worrying about this, caused myself pain, and missed out on some great times as a result of an illusion in my mind.

Now for those of you saying, "well that's easy for you to say, you got a good mark," I would point to several of my friends who didn't get good marks. And are all living successful lives.

What I had pictured as a 10/10 disaster was in reality for those who experienced it, a 2/10 disappointment. So even if what I feared had happened, the consequences weren't what I feared they would be.

The problem is that when we worry, we are not in control of our minds. And when you're not in control, your ego can pull out its full bag of tricks to scare the crap out of you; to feed you endless terrible illusions.

These thoughts get traction because your ego is brilliant at feeding you scenarios that *while incredibly unlikely are not impossible*. So you cannot completely dismiss them, despite the fact that they are highly exaggerated, unlikely, and often borderline preposterous.

The fact that the very distant possibility remains is usually enough for your ego to *turn an unlikely, implausible scenario into the fear that dominates your mind*.

Your mind becomes dominated by chaotic thoughts that create more and ever-bigger worries until checked by structured, accurate thinking. This is why there is absolutely nothing more important than control of your mind.

This is why your fears are not to be trusted. They aren't facts; they are negative illusions.

SIDE NOTE

Have you been practicing the 15 seconds of positive thought and No Mind? I will tell you again what Andy told me: this is the single most important skill you can and ever will gain in life.

I have told you that nothing (and I mean nothing) has had a more profound impact on my life and the lives of those who have learned, practiced, and then mastered this skill. I have told you that without mastering this skill, nothing else I or anyone teaches you will benefit you in the way it could.

And I have told you that Tim Ferriss has called this the meta-skill, the skill that makes all others effective.

If after reading and understanding that, you haven't focused on learning this skill, ask yourself why. Ask yourself if you do want to create the life you dream of; if you do want to be naturally confident and successful; if you do want to become one of the 1% who live life on their terms and are able to reward themselves and those they love with a quality of life that few others can imagine.

So, if that is what you truly desire, then put this book down now and go and practice this skill and keep going until you can hold the 15 seconds of thought and bring in No Mind. Otherwise, you are simply allowing your ego to give you the illusion of progress by continuing to read to the end of this book.

You will feel you have learned lots of great stuff. Your ego will convince you that you now have all the answers; it will tell you that you know things because you've read them. You will probably feel great for a while, but soon enough you will drift back to your old ways of thinking.

It will distract you from the fact that you don't know this at all because you haven't applied the most important lessons and learned the most important skill – control of the tool that dictates all of your success or failure in life. Your mind.

JUST A SITUATION TO DEAL WITH

So when a worry comes up, you need to catch that thought, by observing it instead of judging it, and then use structured, accurate thoughts to re-engage your natural success and confidence mindset.

This allows you to turn that something that harms you (a worry) into something that helps you (an approach to deal with the situation you are actually facing).

The first step is to slow down and get in control of your mind.

The second step is to look at the situation itself, not all the negative illusions and terrible consequences your ego feeds you about the situation. I'll come on to how to deal with those shortly.

For now, just separate out the situation from the consequences, the situation from the illusion. This takes a little practice but is incredibly powerful once you start doing it.

Next, every time your mind, your ego, feeds you a worry thought, simply replace that unhelpful, chaotic thought with the structured thought of:

"This is just a situation to deal with."

When you think this thought instead of worry, you shift from feeling powerless to being in charge; from feeling out of control and at the mercy of events to recognizing the truth that you have an incredible array of tools, options, and choices at your disposal to deal with pretty much every situation you will ever face.

Your dominant thoughts shift from fear and worry to examining how you will deal with the situation you face. Can you feel the shift within you as you simply say to yourself, "This is just a situation to deal with"?

Let me give you an example of how this works with a situation I faced a few years ago.

I had badly ruptured my Achilles tendon playing football. It was a full rupture, which means that there was a big gap in the tendon.

The first consultant I saw decided against surgery despite my protests and said the tendon simply needed to heal with my leg in a protective boot. I instinctively felt that this was the wrong choice, but (against my instincts) I went ahead with what he recommended.

To cut a long story short, that didn't work out. At all.

After two months in a boot and six months of full-on physiotherapy and rehab, my leg wasn't any better. I could only walk with a lot of pain. I couldn't run and my leg was very swollen and just felt all wrong.

I went back to the consultant who gave me an MRI that showed (no surprise) that the tendon hadn't healed properly – that there was lots of bad tissue and was generally in a pretty terrible state.

I was, to say the least, unimpressed that this was the situation I found myself in, despite requesting a different course of action (surgery) in the first place.

His next words though were on a different scale. He said, "I'm afraid your leg is too badly damaged and the risks of surgery are too great. There's nothing we can do. I'm sorry, but your leg will never get any better. You'll have to learn to adjust to being crippled."

I was 40 years old, had always been very active and sporty, and was suddenly being told that I was crippled for life because of a medical choice that I had fought hard against having in the first place.

Now fortunately I had already regained a degree of control over my mind at this stage.

Now the problem I was facing was clearly pretty big. It was clearly very important to me that I got the outcome I desired, which was to not be crippled and to get back full use of my leg.

I think it's fair to say that most people would have been very worried and fearful in that situation. But thanks to having the right way of thinking in place, I wasn't. Don't get me wrong, I wasn't happy about the situation but there was no fear or worry.

Here's what happened in my mind.

I felt the worry thoughts start to emerge. I took a few moments to get back in control of my mind, to ensure that I used the supercomputer between my ears to help me instead of working against me.

I separated out the truth of the situation which was that one consultant (and only one) had told me that nothing could be done. That was an opinion and not a fact.

That meant that all the disaster scenarios were not simply unhelpful but were, at this stage at least, irrelevant. They were excess baggage that would get in the way of me finding the right path forward.

I decided to go for a long drive, to gather my thoughts, to take some time to look at the problem and decide on my course of action.

I knew that after looking at my options and once I had decided on my course of action, that I would apply it. I would see clearly in my mind the outcome I desired and would work diligently, in a workmanlike way towards that outcome. I would focus on the next step that I needed to do and only the next step. I wouldn't move on to the following step until I had completed the one I was on.

I knew I would do everything in my power to achieve the outcome I desired. I accepted that it might take a number of attempts and take some time but I knew that I had a lot of moves to make to get the result to fall my way.

I would find the best solution available, apply it, and wait for the result. I would deal with each level of the problem as it occurred, not all at once. I would do this logically, with my mind clear of all the noise and negative thoughts my ego would seek to throw at me. I would stay focused on the outcome I desired and not get distracted by all the things that could happen, might happen, may happen *but hadn't happened*.

If that wasn't enough, then it wasn't enough and I would accept that meant that I would not achieve the outcome I desired and I would move on after drawing all the lessons, all the value and benefits I could from the situation. I would even be grateful for the growth, experience, strength, and wisdom I would gain from having this experience in my life.

To quote my friend Andy Shaw:

If I lose, I go forward armed with a stronger defense. If I win, I go forward armed with a stronger defense and another victory under my belt. So I either win or I win big: either way I win.

My course of action was to find the best Achilles surgeon I could, and to get the best understanding of the real state of my leg and the options available to me. I accepted that I may need to go through several experts before I found one with the answers I wanted.

On the way home, I remembered (or rather my subconscious served up to me) that David Beckham, the soccer player, had ruptured his Achilles and had had successful treatment and returned to playing football at the elite level.

Instantly my ego told me that any appointment/treatment with the surgeon that treated David Beckham wouldn't be available to a "normal" person like me, would cost too much. I knew, thanks to being in control of my mind, to ignore my ego: it was once again <u>trying to block off possible answers that I hadn't even explored</u>.

I got home and used Google to find the name of the surgeon that operated on David Beckham. I found his name and the hospital he worked in within a few minutes. I did some research on him and he was very clearly the world's leading expert on Achilles injuries and trusted by all the top sports people to treat them. So, I had clearly found a genuine expert.

I called up the hospital in Finland where the surgeon worked (while my ego continued to try to tell me that it would be too expensive) and asked if I could book an appointment with him. Immediately the answer (in perfect English) was, "Yes, no problem, he can see you next week."

How much would the consultation be? The response: 180 euros.

So now, I knew I could see the world's top expert on exactly my injury for 180 euros, within a week. And I got to go to Finland, a place I love.

I had the appointment and he spent a few minutes examining me and a few minutes reviewing the scans of my injury. This was our conversation:

Me: "Can you fix my leg?"

Him: "Yes, no problem."

Me: "So I'm not crippled for life then?"

Him: "No."

Me: "Will I be able to play sport again?"

Him: "Almost certainly."

Me: "Is it a big operation?"

Him: "It will take me about 30 minutes to fix it and you'll be back and running within a few months."

Me: "How much will the operation cost?" (My ego immediately tells me it will be tens of thousands.)

Him: "Five thousand euros."

Me: "When can we do the operation?"

Him: "Next Thursday, if you can make it."

So, for 180 euros I got to see the best Achilles surgeon in the world. Within five minutes, he had told me not only that I wasn't crippled for life but that I could return to playing sport – and it would cost me a fraction of what I had feared.

Can you see that by staying in control of my mind, I was able to separate out the actual situation (one surgeon telling me I was crippled) from the illusions that my ego was feeding me (that my life as I knew it was over; that I would never be able to play properly with my kids; that I would never play sport again)?

And then by unemotionally and without any of the limitations and worries that my ego wanted to push onto me, I was able to focus on finding and then applying the best course of action available to me. And I was able to use the power of my subconscious mind to find an incredible solution.

Can you see how worry and fear would have clouded, blocked, and held back those answers that were there and available to me?

VISIT THE WORST-CASE SCENARIO

One of the things that allows our ego to run riot and create all the fear and anxiety are all the "what ifs?" *The sense that there is no limit to how badly things could go wrong.*

But what if rather than shying away from looking at the very worst-case scenario, you instead fully explored it to see what it would really mean, as opposed to what you <u>fear it might mean</u>?

Because once you've truly explored and understood the limits of what might happen and what you would do if that situation came to pass, there is nothing left to fear. *There are only scenarios that you've already decided how you'll deal with.*

This is the adult equivalent of turning the bedroom light on when you were scared of the monsters under the bed. As soon as you turned the light on you saw the noises or shadows that scared you weren't the monsters you imagined.

You saw the limits to your fears, by the simple act of turning on the light.

And you start to see that while you may not like those scenarios, while they may not be what you would choose, <u>you can see</u> how you would manage them and soon enough thrive off of them, albeit in a different way than you may have planned.

So, take something that you are worried about right now. Allow yourself to explore fully the very worst-case scenario you can see happening. And then consider (just consider) what you would do should that situation come to pass.

Every time I do this, I see that I will be completely OK whether my 3/10 or my 10/10 scenario happens. *I become prepared for them, instead of scared by them*. I know what they are and I know how I would deal with them.

What is there to fear? Fear would simply get in the way of me getting the very best outcome.

TOO GOOD TO BE TRUE VS TOO BAD TO BE TRUE

Have you ever noticed how easily your mind dismisses scenarios that are "**too good to be true**," that are "unrealistically" good, but rarely does the same for scenarios that are *too bad to be true*?

Until your raise your consciousness and elevate your thinking, your ego looks at all the best, most positive, wonderful scenarios that could happen and shows you the reasons that these things are unrealistic and unlikely. And so, there is *no point in getting excited and happy about them*. The realistic possibility of those good things happening as a result is discounted by 99% of people.

Yet our egos never tell us that things are too bad to be true; that they are too bad to be realistic; that they are *so unlikely as to not be worth worrying about*.

We have been taught the lie that we should be cynical and discount all the good things, that this makes us "realistic," grown up, hardheaded, and sensible.

Yet the same thinking cannot be applied to the bad, negative, horror story outcomes. Our egos say that we should prepare for the worst possible outcome, that somehow expecting the worst outcome is realistic and will keep you safe.

So, discount any meaningful possibility of the best outcome and entirely expect the very worst. That's the messed-up definition of being realistic according to 99% of people.

But when you stop and look at it, when you actually examine the evidence of your own life, it isn't actually realistic or accurate at all.

Think back on your own life. How many times has the very worst thing, that nightmare that your ego broadcast to you over and over while you laid awake in bed at 3 a.m. stressing about, how often did that actually happen?

Can you even remember? And even when it did happen, how often was it actually as bad as your ego said it would be?

Well, a study was done on this and it shows just how unnecessary worrying really is.

Over an extended period of time the subjects in the study were asked to write down their worries and then identify which of their misfortunes happened and didn't happen.

The answer?

85% of them didn't happen.

But just as importantly, of the 15% that did happen, 79% of subjects responded that they could handle the difficulty better than expected and that the difficulty actually taught them a lesson.

That means that around 97% of what you worry about is nothing more than your fearful mind punishing you with exaggerations and misperceptions.

Don't let your ego speed you past that last sentence. Slow down and consider what that means for your life.

Worrying is a pointless waste of time 97% of the time.

And bluntly I would argue that for the remaining 3% of the time, the respondents hadn't looked hard enough for the benefit or it simply hadn't appeared yet.

Despite this, nearly everyone spends nearly their whole time worry about something.

The loss of true living, the impact on the quality of life of so many people is staggering – ***based on something that is proven to not be true***.

This is just something for you to think about next time your ego tries to get you to worry.

LIFE IS ALWAYS ON YOUR SIDE

But here is the single biggest reason that you never need to worry again.

Life is always on your side.

The things you worry about, the things you are scared of, if they happen, are in fact gifts. They are life giving you exactly what you need in order to become the greatest version of yourself and to create the life you want to live.

It's just that by judging something as good or bad, you block the good that life/God/the universe (use whatever label works for you) is providing you because it hasn't come in the expected form.

Whether it's something as small as being late for an important appointment or something big like divorce or the prospect of losing your job.

Are you able to master the situation by remaining poised, balanced, in control, and completely unshakable? Or do you get swept up in fear, anxiety, and maybe even start catastrophizing what may happen?

The truth is very few people master remaining calm. Not because they cannot – anyone can learn this – but because they don't look at the "bad" situation in the right way.

Their default thinking is to tumble down the rabbit hole of considering all the terrible consequences, all the pain, anger, resentment, misery, and unhappiness that this situation could lead to.

That's **COULD** lead to, not **WILL** lead to.

It isn't accurate thinking (which is what all good analysis needs). It is negative thinking, falsely labelled as being realistic.

But the 1% who remain completely unshakable no matter what see the world very differently. And as a result, they stay calm naturally and without effort.

Instead of using their minds to look at all the ways things could work out badly, they instead look at all the ways things could work out well. Right now, your ego will probably be screaming that I need to get "real," **but negativity isn't realistic no matter how many people say it is.**

They feed their minds with all the possible ways that this situation could work out for the best for them – not definitely will, just could. They look at all the ways the problem could resolve itself.

They focus on possibilities instead of consequences. And then in a workmanlike way, they move forward with creating the outcome they would most like to see.

But they accept that whatever outcome happens will work out for the best for them. And so, there is nothing to fear, nothing to get anxious about.

It is simply that their highest good has come disguised as something that they didn't want.

It is your judgement of something as bad that stops you being calm, and blocks the incredible gifts life is giving you.

Life is on your side. It always has been and it always will be.

I followed this exact process as I was going through my divorce. My ego had all the material it needed to throw mountains of shit at me, non-stop.

I decided one morning to literally grab a cup of coffee, sit down, and get everything out of my head and shine a very bright light onto all the bullshit my ego was looking to smash me with.

I went through all the what ifs, all the scenarios, all the catastrophes that my ego was using. I worked through everything that might or could happen.

I saw that it was possible that I would only get to see my children every other weekend which was absolutely not what I wanted. I did not want to be in any way distant from my daughters who are my world.

I had seen close friends get alienated from their children after a divorce through no fault of their own and some had missed out on years of their children's lives, some forever.

My ego beat me up with the idea that I would not be able to be there for my children when they needed me, that something would happen and I would not be there to protect them. I was concerned that any future partner of my ex-wife could be unkind, aggressive, or abusive towards my daughters. And if I was alienated from them or had limited access to them, again my ability to protect them was compromised.

I saw the possibility of me having to pay my ex-wife a material proportion of my income, which alongside the possibility of limited access to my children meant I would effectively be forced to pay for a situation which I felt would be completely wrong and utterly against the best interests of my daughters.

I saw that I would be at best going a very long way backwards financially: that I would be worse off than I was when I met my wife; that, despite a marriage that had only in reality lasted a few years, I would have to pay over half of my wealth. The wealth that I had built up prior to meeting her would be lost.

I saw that I may lose my home, **my daughter's home**. I saw that they may have to leave their school, as the legal costs continued to mount up.

I saw that I may go bankrupt as the legal costs stacked up and I could fall behind on the payments I needed to make on my mortgage, credit cards, etc. And that this would leave me in a less strong position to fight to get the best possible outcome from the divorce itself.

There were many, many more but you get the picture – losing my kids, going bankrupt, paying out what little I had to my ex-wife.

I went and experienced each of these scenarios. I accepted and surrendered to the fact that they could happen, that they were possible outcomes.

But I also then refocused my mind to see that however much I didn't want each and every one of those scenarios, that if they came to pass, they would ultimately be for the best – even if there was no way I could see that at the time.

I saw that no matter what I would never stop fighting to get equal access to my children. I would make sure they knew that I never stopped fighting to be with them no matter what. I saw that this would likely strengthen rather than weaken our bond in the long term.

I saw that if they lost their home and went to a different school, that this was the perfect opportunity to teach them everything I had learned about mindset, confidence, and resilience and how they would grow massively stronger as a result.

I saw that even the worst possible financial outcome would provide me with the incredible inspiration to break through any barriers that could have otherwise held me back to create the business success I desired. It meant I knew I would turn *Unstoppable Self-Confidence* into a huge success.

After spending some time working through the possibilities instead of simply dwelling on the consequences, I felt a complete sense of peace about the outcome. I knew what I desired. I knew I would do everything in my power to bring about the outcome I was after. But I knew either way that things would be absolutely fine.

I then saw my ego's fears in the cold light of day and **calibrated my view of them accurately.** I saw then that my current lens on those fears was a 10/10 disaster scenario. I saw that the most likely outcome was that I would get fair access to my children, that we would resolve the divorce, and that if it went to court, I was in a strong position anyway.

I saw that the likely worst-case scenario was a 3/10 not a 10/10.

Now here's what's incredibly powerful about this.

By doing this, by accepting and surrendering to the outcome no matter what it was, I completely took away my ego's power to cause me pain, to put me into fear, worry, or anxiety. After all, I had already visited in my mind the dark places it was trying to take me. I had already seen how not only would I survive that scenario, but how it would work out for the best for me.

That meant I was incredibly mentally strong without any effort. I didn't need to try to be strong, to try not to be scared. I simply wasn't. It took no effort at all.

Even better, all that mental energy that would have otherwise been wasted on processing disaster scenarios or dealing with worry, fear, and anxiety was now freed up to focus on finding the answers that would lead me to the outcome I wanted.

I was no longer handicapped by having half my energy being used on pointless fear and worry.

Despite what the world thinks, this is your natural way of operating. It isn't natural to dwell, to soak in your fears and anxieties. Your natural way is to simply deal with the situations life presents you with, take the benefits, leave the baggage, and grow.

One of the most important things Stephen ever told me was that I should embrace my problems; that they were in fact my friends, showing me what I needed to learn in order to become who I wanted to be and to create my life on my terms.

And once I understood this, I would realize the truth that there was no need to be fearful or anxious. I simply needed to see that life was always on my side.

THINGS TO CONSIDER

- Can you imagine what your life would look like if you eliminated worry from your life? Can you imagine what it would feel like to never need to worry again?

- Have you fallen for the mind trap that you "should" worry? That it is "responsible" to worry? That being fearful or worrying somehow keeps you safe?

- Consider: How does worrying about anything help you? Could you simply choose to be aware and conscious of what could happen instead?

- Can you see how worrying is causing yourself pain about something that might happen? Can you see how it's causing you pain based on an illusion without the problem actually needing to exist?

- Can you see how being in a state of fear or worry switches off your incredible subconscious minds' ability to solve problems?

- Consider how you get more of what you focus on. So, the more your dominant thoughts are about fears and worries, the more you will get things to worry about and fear.

- Do you focus on possibility or consequence? Understanding the difference that this focus makes to your life, where do you want to focus your thinking now?

- Consider that each fear is a limit on your life. How many limits (fears) do you want to accept from now on?

- Consider that the things you fear are just "situations to be dealt with."

- Consider that life is always on your side; that life always works out for the best even when it comes disguised as something bad. It is only your judgement of something as good or bad that blocks you from receiving the gifts you are being given.

CHAPTER 10

UNINSTALLING
NEGATIVITY

> **Do not allow negative thoughts into your mind for they are the weeds that strangle confidence.**
>
> BRUCE LEE

Your life is a reflection of your thinking.

Despite knowing this truth, the vast majority of the world spends most of their time thinking predominantly negative thoughts. But more than that, they soak in their negativity.

They focus on their problems instead of their possibilities; on what's wrong instead of all the things they could be grateful for; on lack instead of abundance; and on their fears instead of their dreams.

Like the other layers of backwards, muddled thinking I've talked about in this book, this is something that they learned. It isn't a natural way to think.

Negativity is a virus. It spreads almost uncontrollably from one person to the next through the news, social media, and day-to-day interactions. As more and more people become infected it becomes seen as normal even though it is anything but. Just because most of the world does something insane, that doesn't make it "normal."

Unless you've taken steps to consciously protect and guard your mind against this virus, you are likely to have been hurt by it too.

Here's how a person becomes infected and then "taken down" by negativity.

Through interaction with someone negative or through exposure to negativity on the news or social media, etc., you begin to become aware of the bad things that could happen – of the negative, nasty ways that some people behave or the bad things that sometimes happen in the world.

These negative things aren't the sum total of the human experience or even a vaguely accurate reflection of it. But they are the ones that prey on our fears and so most easily capture our attention.

If you interact with negativity enough of the time (through regular use of social media, 24-hour "news" networks, regular interaction with negative people), <u>awareness</u> of the "bad stuff" turns into <u>expecting</u> the bad stuff. As soon as you switch from awareness to expectation, you're infected with the negativity virus.

Once infected, you begin to see the world differently and subtle shifts in your focus from seeing the good to searching for the bad start to take place.

Whenever something "bad" happened, you felt smart, like you were now aware of the "real world" that was really out there. You're no longer naïve, like you had been before, thinking that the world was a good and decent place.

You now know the (negative) "truth."

You got persuaded that it was right to scan the horizon for all the bad things that could happen and "probably would." You came to expect them.

And when after enough searching you found things that were "wrong," this simply confirmed your view that you were right to be cynical – that this kept you prepared, safe from harm, and protected in some way.

You continued to train your mind to focus on the negative and you discovered more and more things to feel negative about, all "good evidence" that reinforced your new negative view of the world.

Soon enough, this way of thinking wasn't simply a habit – it became your default setting. When faced with any new scenario your first thoughts became:

- What will go wrong with this?
- How will I get screwed over by this?
- Who will let me down next?

Because your dominant thoughts were negative, maybe even cynical, your subconscious mind sought out evermore data and "evidence" to align with that view. And in the process, it filtered out all the data and evidence that challenged that view. Remember that your mind, *through confirmation bias*, seeks out evidence to support and align with your dominant thoughts and filters out evidence that contradicts them.

Soon enough you become addicted to negativity, to a small or large extent. But if you expect things to go wrong, to be let down or disappointed, negativity has caught you too.

Negativity eventually *becomes part of your identity* which means that your ego (which always looks to keep you stuck exactly where you are) fights any attempt to let it go. Now negativity is no longer a choice, it's part of who you are. And to change means losing part of who you are.

THE UNSEEN DAMAGE OF A NEGATIVE MINDSET

The damage caused by a negative mindset is horrific. It is insidious. It slowly eats away at your confidence and success mindset until it destroys your ability to create the life you want to live.

It's almost uniquely toxic because it presents itself as a way of keeping you safe. In that way it acts like a Trojan horse virus, creeping inside your defenses by acting as a friend, then once inside, unleashing a war against you.

Your ego uses negativity to keep you stuck, by telling you that it is keeping you safe from harm; that you are being smart by keeping your defenses up, when in fact the barriers it constructs block your growth and success.

When you break up with a partner, it tells you things like you should never let anyone get close to you again, to protect yourself from that pain. It doesn't tell you that you've just turned <u>temporary pain</u> that is designed to help you learn what a good partner looks like, into <u>permanent pain</u> that will compromise any future relationship.

If you fail in business, your ego uses the negative mindset to tell you that the pain and loss or failure (which is designed to help you learn what you need to achieve your dreams and desires) is something to be avoided at all costs – because "you've already tried that once and it didn't work."

It doesn't tell you that the decision not to try again guarantees your permanent failure in life and stops you from applying the incredible lessons you could otherwise learn from your failure – lessons which, if applied, would guarantee your future success.

None of this keeps you safe at all. It simply keeps you stuck and blocked from the thoughts and actions that would create the life you want.

The truth of course is that negativity does not work and does not deliver any real benefit to us.

Negativity doesn't help you avoid the bad outcome, it creates it.

Here's how this works.

Negative thoughts create negative emotions which in turn produce negative actions. Those negative actions create more things to feel negative about and so the cycle repeats and a negative, downward spiral is created.

Our minds are perceptual machines. This means that our minds are filters, filtering in and out of our conscious awareness the things that are most relevant to us.

How is what's most relevant defined? By your dominant thoughts.

So if your dominant thoughts are focused on your problems, on all the things that are wrong in your life, your subconscious mind, the most powerful machine in the known universe, sets out to find more and more things that are wrong and to present them to you.

So your life fills up with evermore problems.

Whereas if your dominant thoughts are on all the things that you have to be grateful and thankful for, your subconscious mind takes <u>that</u> instruction and finds evermore things to fill your life with that you will be grateful for.

We communicate, we <u>instruct</u> our subconscious minds, through our dominant thoughts and feelings – not by the words we use. That is why most people accidently create bad stuff in their lives when they desire good stuff.

That's why focusing on what you're grateful for isn't just some woo-woo, new age hippie thing.

It's how you get what you want, on purpose, using your incredible subconscious mind to work for you instead of accidentally against you.

WEIGHING YOU DOWN ON YOUR JOURNEY

Remember, no thought stands still. Every single thought you ever have either helps you or harms you. So what's the harm done by negative thought?

Well, every single negative thought (yes, every single one) comes with a cost. You may not immediately see the cost, but it's there. You may simply have never taken the time to consider it.

Andy once told me to imagine every single negative thought as a piece of baggage that you pick up and carry with you on your journey through life; not useful baggage with all the essentials that you need to speed you on your way to your destination; not the lessons and benefits from everything you've experienced and gone through; not all the value.

This is pointless baggage, heavy, difficult to carry, and uncomfortable.

The more baggage you pick up, the slower your journey and the less energy you have to move forward. Pick up enough baggage and soon enough you won't be moving forward at all.

Your journey will stop.

And you won't be able to make any progress until you shed some of the dead weight. If you're not yet the person you want to be and you're not yet living the life you want to live, then this is you.

All of this costs you your ability to create, your ability to grow and progress. It means you are investing your energy in processing the past, not in creating the future. It keeps you stuck, not moving forward.

If you've had a shitty relationship with a former partner, a parent, a sibling, or friend and have anger and resentment about the way you were treated, then this is holding you back from creating future relationships that would benefit you.

If you were bullied at school or at work, had a pain-in-the-ass boss who treated you like shit, <u>that resentment and anger</u> will at best distract you and at worst block you from doing the things you need to do to create the life you want and from interacting with people in ways that help you.

If through the cumulative weight of "bad" experiences you have become cynical and <u>expect to be let down</u>, disappointed, or mistreated, this means that you have, in effect, given up on your ability to create the life you want.

If you spend your life in fear, worry, anxiety, or doubt, this will take up huge amounts of your creative and emotional energy – energy that could have otherwise been used to create the life you want and to become the person you want to be.

Imagine how far you could go and how much more quickly you could get there if you put down this baggage; if your energy was focused on enjoying the present and creating the future rather than reliving the pain of the past.

Do you think you'd make more progress?

Take a few moments to consider what baggage you are carrying with you. Consider how much of that baggage is useful to you and how much is simply weighing you down.

Remember, you're in control. So any time you like, you can choose to put down the baggage you no longer need.

THE PROBLEM WITH THE BLAME GAME

When you blame others, you give up your power to change.

– DR ROBERT ANTHONY

How much do you blame and criticize others? How much do you consider other people, outside events and circumstances to be responsible for the state of your life today?

For how you feel, and for what you have achieved and not achieved? For the bad things that have happened to you?

Blame is incredibly seductive. When we blame others or outside events, we absolve ourselves of responsibility for what has happened. It means we are not at fault and at a deeper level we think it means that there is nothing wrong with us. Most people fear blame and being wrong for the same reasons they fear mistakes.

They identify with the problem, so it becomes something they are, not simply something they did.

What I mean by this is that when something "bad" happens or something goes wrong, you can choose to see it as an event, as just something that happened. Or you can choose to see that event as in some way revealing something about you and who you are.

One is the fixed mindset approach and the other is the growth mindset approach. If you see the "bad" thing as just an event, you are using a growth mindset and **then the event becomes research, something to draw lessons from so that you can go forward better, strong, and wiser.**

If you see the event through a fixed mindset then every mistake becomes an existential threat, an emotional threat to your self-esteem and well-being, not simply something that occurred and an experience to learn from.

And so most people rush to blame others, to broadcast to the world and more importantly to themselves, "Look, there's nothing wrong with me. I'm not faulty, I'm not inadequate."

And they feel better in the moment because they feel that they've dealt with the threat to their identity. But they've missed the opportunity life was giving them to learn and grow.

As soon as you decide someone else is to blame, you've told yourself that there is nothing for you to learn.

And so, the opportunity to grow and develop, to become more, to get wiser, is lost.

The problem is that <u>blaming others is excusing yourself</u> – excusing yourself from learning every lesson you can, and excusing yourself from becoming the very best version of yourself you can be.

THE POWER OF TAKING 100% RESPONSIBILITY FOR EVERYTHING

There is a very different choice available to you. It's a choice that sets you free but comes disguised as one that puts you in the firing line.

Imagine giving up the need to ever blame anyone or anything ever again. *No matter what.* No matter what someone else did, no matter what circumstances you faced, imagine taking 100%, complete responsibility for everything.

Imagine giving up the need to even avoid being blamed for anything again.

No more wasted conversation about who should have done what, who was right, and who was wrong.

Well, you are 100% responsible for your life.

Note that I didn't say 100% in control. I said 100% responsible – there's a difference.

What that means is that the success, the quality of your life, is almost entirely based on your response to the situations and circumstances you face, not the situations or circumstances themselves.

Each time something happens in your life, no matter how good, bad, or indifferent it is, you face a choice.

That choice is, "Who do I choose to be in this situation? How do I choose to respond to the situation I face?"

Every time you choose to respond in a way that aligns with your design of the best version of yourself, you win. You empower yourself; you make the choice to grow and to become stronger, better, and wiser. You extract the maximum value from every situation.

Each time you don't choose this, each time you blame others for where you are and who you've become, you lose. You lose your power to change; you disempower yourself from making new choices; you make yourself a victim and at the mercy of situations or events.

One choice helps you, the other harms you.

WOULD YOU RATHER BE RIGHT OR HAPPY?

No one to blame. That was why most people led lives
they hated, with people they hated. How wonderful to
have someone to blame! How wonderful to live with one's
nemesis. You may be miserable, but you feel forever in the

right. You may be fragmented, but you feel absolved of all the blame for it. Take your life in your own hands and what happens? A terrible thing: no-one to blame.

– ERICA JONG

So, would you rather be right or would you rather be happy?

This question strikes at the very core of blame culture. Most people choose, consciously or unconsciously, to be "right," to not be blamed. Their emotional need to not "be in the wrong" becomes their focus.

They focus on not losing the argument instead of winning in their life.

There's an old saying of be careful of winning the battle but losing the war – which is exactly what happens when you allow blame into your life.

Let me give you an example.

At the start of my divorce, I felt a lot of anger, resentment, and blame towards my ex-wife. This is obviously a very common, "normal" way to feel in a divorce and in any relationship breakup. I spent a lot of time talking this through with Stephen, the brilliant coach that helped me figure out a lot of what is in this book.

His work, very early on in our sessions, was to shift my thinking away from any thoughts of blaming my ex-wife. He showed me that I could spend all of my sessions with him talking through all the things that my ex-wife had done that made me angry, resentful, or upset. In some of those situations those feelings would be "justified"; in others, not so much.

But the certain outcome was that at the end of our sessions, my life wouldn't have taken a single step further forward. I could explain to Stephen how "right" I was in all of this; how bad I felt my ex-wife's behavior had been; how wrong she was.

But what would I learn from that? How would that make my life better now or in the future? How would it help my daughters?

My ex-wife was no doubt feeling similar feelings towards me, based on our different perspectives of what had happened.

Let's assume, purely to illustrate this point, that I was 100% in the right and she was 100% in the wrong. That meant I had literally nothing to learn, no value to gain, no growth, wisdom, or experience to extract from this situation. All opportunity to change and grow, gone.

Did I really think that was true? Is that who I wanted to be in this situation? How would that judgement (be careful of that word!) leave me in any better position for my next relationship?

Stephen explained that when people get stuck, when they get addicted to blaming others, they get locked into a destructive pattern of behavior. Through blaming, they start to create and then stack resentments towards their partner. And if I didn't resolve this pattern, I would take it into my next relationship.

The resentment stacking creates a negative mindset and this can trigger the person to look for more problems in the relationship. A person looking for problems is always going to find something negative; and when they find it, they can resent that too.

Over time those resentments can become overwhelming, leading the person to want to stop the pain, the pain they associate with their partner. They will start to put up walls to protect themselves from their partner.

This is a lethal combination of emotions for any relationship. If one partner feels that they have to protect themselves from the other, how can they keep their love alive? There is a real danger that they will turn off any feelings that they have towards their partner and that they will retreat to a detached or numb emotional state.

But the problem is that when you turn off the bad feelings towards your partner, you turn off the good ones too. And so, the relationship starts to die.

If the person who is blaming and stacking resentments decides to leave the relationship but carries forward that same pattern of blaming and resentment, the pattern will simply repeat itself.

Over and over in relationships, they will convince themselves that they were right, that they didn't meet the right person, that marriage or relationships don't work.

They will never see their own destructive behavior pattern and its contribution to the pain and downfall of their relationships. They will remain unhappily "right," instead of challenging themselves; instead of learning and growing, and so, maximizing their own happiness.

THE PROBLEM WITH PLAYING THE VICTIM

The victim mindset dilutes the human potential. By not accepting personal responsibility for our circumstances, we greatly reduce the power to change them.

– DR STEVE MARABOLI

When you continue to blame, to externalize responsibility for your life, what you're telling yourself is that you are essentially powerless. After all, if all of the bad things in your life happen **to you** not **by you**, then any happiness, confidence, or success could get taken away at any moment, by anyone or anything.

Can you see how disempowering this way of thinking is? How blame, which looks like strength, is actually a huge weakness in disguise?

The choice lies in whether you see yourself as a victim of your circumstances or a product of your decisions. That choice determines your ability to create the life you want and to be who you want to be.

You cannot be a victim and a success at the same time.

And no matter what anyone tells you it's always a choice: a choice to get stronger, wiser, and better every day no matter your circumstances.

The 1% who live life on their terms have as much bad shit happen to them as anyone else. The difference is that they never allow themselves to become victims because they know that this is one of the most damaging, toxic mindsets you can ever have.

At its core, the victim mentality is disempowering, weak, and creates a sense of helplessness that destroys your ability to live a successful, happy, confident life.

It says that you have no meaningful responsibility for who you are or what your life has become. There are few better ways of creating a big downward spiral in your life than by playing the victim.

Confident, successful people know that they are in charge of their life. They refuse to allow themselves or their lives to be defined by anything other than themselves. When something happens, instead of feeling negative, helpless, or looking for someone to blame, they immediately look for the path forward, the lessons to learn, and the path to grow from the experience.

They look to win from each and every experience they face. Sometimes they win and sometimes they win big. But they decide; *they choose* to always win.

They know that they can allow their focus to drift and indulge the bad, or they can sharpen their focus on the good, on the lessons.

Confident, successful people always, no matter what, look for the value and the benefit and drop anything else. They do not pick up another piece of baggage that will weigh them down and make their journey harder or longer.

Remember, you are 100% responsible, not 100% in control.

Same circumstances, different mindsets, leading to very different outcomes. One makes you weaker no matter what; the other makes you unstoppable.

OVERCOMING THE FEELING OF POWERLESSNESS

A lot of negative feelings really come from feeling powerless. After all, if you *knew* you had the power to change the situation or circumstances you face you would just go ahead and do it.

But if you feel powerless, unable to influence or change the situation you face, you lapse into complaining about it, bitching about it rather than *doing something* about it.

But this feeling of powerlessness is an illusion, a lie told to you by your ego to keep you stuck and playing small.

How often have you given away your power and chosen helplessness instead? How often have you told yourself that you "have" to do something instead of reminding yourself of the truth that you are *choosing* to do something?

Most people (and in the past, I've done this more than I'd like to admit) choose to say that they "can't," that they "have no choice," that they "have to."

They find it easier to tell themselves that comfortable lie rather than face the uncomfortable but empowering truth: *that you always have a choice.*

That choice may not be easy, and you may not like the consequences, but it remains a choice nonetheless. On rare, specific occasions the consequences of a decision may be such that you don't make what looks like your ideal choice.

But most people are masters at turning "don't want to" into "have no choice."

They choose to weaken themselves time and again by giving into negative comments, guilt trips, pressure from friends, peers, teachers, criticism from others, and not being clear about their boundaries.

As long as you allow other people to have a negative influence over the way you think, feel, and behave, you'll struggle to live life on your terms. Their negativity will infect you and drag you down.

Giving away your power is a choice, and one that will erode your self-esteem, the self-esteem that can only come from you feeling in charge of your own life.

The antidote is to become conscious of your thoughts. Each time you tell yourself in any way that you have no choice, slow down and consider if that's really true.

Remind yourself of the truth *that you are the decider in your life*, and that your choice is to make decisions that align with you living as the person you want to be.

You are not powerless. you are the decider in your life. See how different life feels from that one simple change.

DEALING WITH NEGATIVE PEOPLE

Do not allow negative people to turn you into one of them.

– ANONYMOUS

There was a guy I used to work with who was probably the most negative-minded person I have ever met.

I generally got into work very early as the office was quiet and I could get my important work done when my head was clear and when there were less people in the office to disturb me. More often than not I was the first one in.

The second person in (we'll call him Chris) was this negative person. I could hear him come in and I swear I could almost feel his negative energy as he came to sit down at the desk near to mine.

Chris loved, *and I mean really loved*, to start off his day with a good moan, a proper complaining and whining session. Even the way he used to sit down was negative.

He used to drop into his chair with a massive sigh, which was the prelude to him starting his moan session. You could tell that his journey into work was his opportunity to collect together all the things he could whine to everyone about as soon as he got into the office.

I swear he used to look forward to it.

As soon as he sat down, he would start to complain and talk to me about all the "awful," "crap," "terrible," "shit" things that were going on. He complained endlessly: about the time taken to get to work and his coffee not being warm enough to the shit meetings he was going to have later that day and all the work he was now going to have to do because everyone else was "fucking useless." He told me how no one understood how hard he worked for little reward, and how much the company would fall apart if it wasn't for all his efforts.

This used to continue for about 30 minutes and as each new person arrived in the office, he would try to bring them into the conversation.

By the end of that 30 minutes, pretty much everyone around him felt a mixture of irritation and wishing he would just stop talking. But everyone felt in some way worse. I would feel slightly poisoned, contaminated by his negativity.

Chris was an energy vampire, someone who, with every interaction, made you feel slightly worse, slightly less OK with the day. Don't me get wrong, he wasn't a bad, nasty, or vindictive person. He was just completely unconscious of his behavior and the impact on those around him.

But the problem was, his identity was tied up in his negativity. More importantly, he got his *significance* and sense of self-worth from his complaining and negativity. Without his daily dose of complaining, his self-esteem would fall away; he didn't know who he was without being negative and complaining. So, he couldn't stop it.

What made him feel significant was the fact that he saw all these "problems" that "no one else did." *So, his behavior followed his significance.*

If you want to understand why anyone does almost anything, look at where they get <u>their significance</u> from. You can then start to understand why they find that (usually destructive) behavior so difficult to change. If being negative, a victim, etc., is what you believe (consciously or unconsciously) makes you significant, makes you matter, you will struggle to give that behavior up, no matter how destructive. It will continue until you find your significance from something else, something better and more worthwhile.

I'm sure you know people like Chris. No doubt you have someone like this that you have to deal with. And it can be very toxic to be around.

I found I would feel irritated or angry as soon as Chris walked into the office, dreading the inevitable tap on my shoulder as he gleefully got ready to unleash his latest rant.

But I soon realized, I reminded myself that I wasn't a victim, I wasn't passive, and that it was my choice whether I put up with this behavior and negativity around me or not. <u>The problem was that I had gone unconscious and given into the lie that I had to tolerate this.</u>

When I snapped back into consciousness and regained control of my mind in that moment, I realized the truth.

I didn't have to tolerate this. I could make a different choice. I could take control of my interactions with him.

So the next morning when Chris was about to start his rant, I calmly, respectfully but very firmly turned to him and said, "Chris – listen. I get in early to concentrate on my work, this time is important to me. You need to let me concentrate."

He looked a little shocked, but it hardly ever happened again. There were a couple of occasions when I needed to reinforce the message, but 95% of the problem was dealt with there and then.

DON'T LISTEN TO THE DREAM STEALERS

There are two types of people who will tell you that you cannot make a difference in this world: those who are afraid to try and those who are afraid you will succeed.

– RAY GOFORTH

One of the most subtle and insidious ways in which people inject their negativity into others is through "helpful" advice. This is negativity disguised as "niceness" and it is one of the most sabotaging, undermining, and damaging forms of negativity.

It is so damaging because it is presented as something well intentioned and helpful, and so it slips in under most people's defenses and destroys their ability to achieve their dreams. But it is sabotage, pure and simple.

This is other people attempting to impose **their false limitations into your mind**.

Those who, by accident or design, seek to keep you playing small and who most often disguise this sabotage as being "realistic" or "protecting you" from "inevitable disappointment."

Those who seek to fill your mind with "helpful" words like, "You won't be able to do that," "You should be realistic," "That's very risky," "What if it doesn't work out," "You might lose money," "You've never done that before," and hundreds more comments just like this.

And those comments nearly always come from people who have never achieved what you are seeking to achieve. So therefore, they are not <u>expert wisdom</u>. They are <u>mere opinions</u> from people with little to zero experience of creating the success you desire.

And the more you progress, the more sabotaging comments you will get. When you hear these comments, slow down, still your mind, and ask yourself one simple question.

Does this comment help me get closer to my goal or does it work against me?

If it doesn't help you, it has to go. Remember from now on you are only interested in things, thoughts, actions, behaviors, and feelings that help you. Everything that works against you is to be dropped.

Your natural success mindset is only interested in value and benefit, not carrying harmful, negative baggage.

Realize the truth that every one of these "helpful" comments are opinions not facts. Like everything else, they should be assessed for value. And they say everything about that person's chances of success, not yours.

How many of the people in your life lift you up and how many drag you down?

How many of them inspire you, encourage you to live the life you dream of, and how many work against you?

Everyone has people in their lives who will sabotage, undermine, resist, manipulate, and criticize them when they try to improve themselves.

Sometimes this is unconscious behavior revealing their own shortcomings and insecurities, but just as often it is entirely on purpose.

Far too often this is the people closest to you, who see your attempts to grow as being a backhanded criticism of them.

Becoming aware of when this sabotage is happening and being clearheaded about how to handle it is crucial for you to live the life you want.

The first question to ask yourself is: Why you would want someone in your life who actively opposes you making your life better?

Take a moment to consider that.

Why would you choose to have people in your life who use their time and energy to find ways, by accident or design, to prevent you from living your dream life?

Imagine how much more progress you would be able to make without them holding you back. Imagine if you only had people in your life who supported and encouraged you to be all you could be.

While this can be painful and challenging to face up to, it is essential to your success.

This doesn't have to mean cutting people out of your life, although sometimes that is necessary.

But it does mean being clear and ruthless about what is and is not acceptable in your life and not tolerating negativity and sabotage from those around you.

HOW TO DEFEAT NEGATIVITY

Nothing in life has any meaning except
the meaning we give it.

– TONY ROBBINS

The antidote to negativity is to avoid judgement, to avoid judging the things in your life as inherently good or bad. This is a false lens on life and one that can stifle your progress and slow you down.

Instead, replace negative thinking and negative judgement with observation and looking for value in any situation. Remember the truth, that life is always on your side, and always gives you exactly what you need to progress to the next level.

In every situation, your job is to look for the lesson, the benefit, so that you can apply it, learn it, and start living at the next level of life.

Negativity stops this process dead in its tracks. Negativity is judgement, the decision that things are bad, won't work, will go wrong, will let you down, and will leave you disappointed.

Negativity means you've lost before you've even started. And so, life needs to repeat the lesson.

The problem with making a judgement is that you stop thinking, stop considering what a situation means. You stop looking for the benefits in the "problem" as soon as you label it a problem and therefore something bad and to be avoided.

You filter out the nuggets of gold that life is giving you, that could well take you to exactly where you've been trying to go, *just in a different way to the way that you planned*.

When what the world calls a "problem" comes up, how about instead of judging it as bad, you simply looked for the possible ways you could benefit from it? This is not to say that you definitely will, only that you could.

This is how, as my friend Richard Wilkins says, you turn your shit into manure.

Imagine if instead of focusing your mind on all the terrible things that could happen to you, you instead focused mainly on the possibilities.

If you searched for the value, the benefit in any situation, how different would your experience of life be?

When dealing with a negative person, use this as practice. You are not judging yourself as superior in any way (there is no value to you in that). Instead, simply use the negative situation or person to observe how well you are able to control your mind, to observe the negativity but not become part of it; to see it and watch it but stay separate.

TAKING 100% RESPONSIBILITY

To get the life you want, you have to take 100% responsibility for your life.

That means giving up on all the reasons you've given yourself for why you're not yet who you want to be or living the life you want to live.

When you blame external circumstances, you become passive and reactive to life. Your mindset becomes weaker as you decide that circumstances determine your success not your choices.

But when you take responsibility for where you are, you empower yourself to make choices that work for you. The truth is that everything you want is a choice.

Confidence is a choice.

Becoming your best self is a choice.

Success is a choice.

Great relationships are a choice.

Wealth is a choice.

You decide who you want to be and how you want your life to look. And then you do whatever is necessary to get to the next step. No matter what has happened to you, someone has faced something tougher and created the life they want. The quality of your life is a choice you make, whether you want to believe that or not.

What choice will you make?

THINGS TO CONSIDER

- Consider: What benefit does negativity have for your life?

- Consider: What negative baggage have you been carrying that you no longer need and that you can now put down?

- Consider, you are 100% responsible for your life – not 100% in control, but 100% responsible.

- Can you see how blaming others is excusing yourself?

- Consider that by focusing on the negative, you simply create more negativity in your life.

- Consider: Would you rather be right or happy?

- Can you see that you always have a choice, that you are the decider in your life?

- Be careful of the "helpful" advice of others which is simply negativity and sabotage in disguise.

- Consider that the antidote to negativity is observation instead of judgement.

FREE GIFT # 2 – BONUS LESSON: "HOW TO ELIMINATE ANY LIMITING BELIEF"

If you'd like to learn the exact steps I use to help people eliminate limiting beliefs (even ones that have held them back for years) – go to **www.unstoppableselfconfidence.com/confidence-on-demand** and watch "How To Eliminate Any Limiting Belief" where I run through this proven process step-by-step. I've also included a free summary crib sheet to help you apply this to your own limiting beliefs. It's absolutely free. Enjoy.

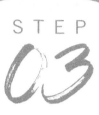
INSTALLING
THE MINDSET
OF THE 1%

CHAPTER 11

RECLAIM YOUR SUPERPOWER: YOUR NATURAL SUCCESS MINDSET

You are a superhero pretending to be an ordinary person.

RICHARD WILKINS

I'd like you to take a moment and do some focused daydreaming.

To open your eyes and, more importantly, your mind to what's **not only possible but probable for you** when you get your thinking right.

To open your mind to **who you can become and what your life can be** when you reconnect with your natural success and confidence mindset.

So, take a few moments, take a breath, and slow down. Bring in your 15 seconds of positive thought (yes, this still matters) and then bring in No Mind.

So, still your mind and when you're ready, read on.

In your mind, picture the person you dream of becoming, the grandest version of the greatest vision you had about yourself and your life.

Really go for this. Take the handbrake off and really dream of who you could be. This is your time to daydream, just like you did when you were a child. There are no limitations here. Ignore any need from your ego to be in any way "realistic" or to figure out whether or how this is possible. You're just daydreaming, so go for it.

Look upon who you have become; see the person you now are in that picture in your mind.

See and, more importantly, feel all the incredible things that you have achieved; see all the incredible, astonishing potential within yourself that you have unleashed, all the greatness within you that you have set free.

See the calmness, the certainty, the serenity that you radiate out.

The calm, clear knowing that no matter what happens, you are fine. The certainty that you can create your life as you desire it to be. *It is simply a process.*

Fear, worry, and anxiety are no longer part of your life. You just calmly deal with whatever you need to deal with on the journey to your inevitable success.

Feel how amazing it feels to have become that person. In your mind, see yourself in the mirror and see how incredible the person looking back at you is. In your mind, look back and review the journey you went on to become that person, to create the incredible life that you have now been living for the last few years.

Soak in this feeling; experience all the details.

All of what you have just experienced is who you really are and the life that is there, ready and waiting for you.

That is the real you, the person you are _destined_ to be. That is your true life, the one you are _destined_ to live.

All you have to do is choose that path and get out of your own way. Remember, you are not capable of having a dream or desire that you are not capable of achieving.

Now you've seen the truth about yourself, maybe for the first time. Will you choose to fulfill that incredible potential?

That is the journey we're about to go on. The exact step-by-step blueprint for you to become that person and create that life.

THE JOURNEY BACK TO CONFIDENCE & SUCCESS

The first step in that journey, and the most critical, was giving you the process to regain control of your mind – the tool you use to create everything in your life, whether good, "bad," or in between.

All success starts with you being in control of your mind. Everything that exists in your life today is a reflection of your thinking and your control of your thinking.

Your ability to choose thoughts that help you, instead of thoughts that work against you is the foundation for getting the life you want on purpose instead of the life you don't, by accident.

By becoming aware of your ego, you see that whenever you think a thought that causes you pain, makes you feel bad, and blocks your success, that isn't you. It's your ego.

By understanding that your ego exists and that the negative voice in your head isn't the real you, you can shift to being the observer of your thoughts. By separating from your thoughts, by observing them instead of being them, you have the power to change them.

When you (incorrectly) think those thoughts *are you*, part of who you are then they limit you. When you realize you can choose your thoughts, your perception of the world, your world, shifts on its axis. Because now you can choose the very best thoughts.

This is the essence of the saying, *"Change your thinking, change your world."*

Your identity shifts from you thinking that you are your ego, to realizing that the real you is entirely separate from your ego. And as a result, who you are and who you can become, becomes open to possibility once again instead of fixed and locked into false limits. Just like when you were a child, *in your natural state*.

This sets the basis for you seeing the core underlying truth of everything that I teach here: *that there's nothing wrong with you and that you don't need fixing*.

That all of those limits, all of that sense of not being good enough, not being capable enough, not being deserving, not being the kind of person who can…is not who you really are.

It never was the truth of who you are and it never will be.

The truth that you have now seen, is that your limits – your lack of success, your lack of confidence, you not yet creating the life you want to live and becoming the person you want to be – is a result of layers and layers of bad teaching, muddled thinking, stifling, limiting social conditioning, and the undermining thoughts of most of society that you came to think were "normal."

These layers of bad programming blocked your natural confidence and success mindset and caused you to become much, much, much less than you are. They caused you to play small, to downplay and dismiss your dreams, and to feel bad about who you are, the way you look, and the thoughts you think.

They caused you, through an appalling education system to get you to uncritically take orders, to not question, to fit in, to give up your voice, and to spend a lifetime seeking the approval and validation of others.

In short, it taught you to work your ass off, spending your precious life living to a blueprint that wasn't yours and never was.

This blueprint can't make you happy and can't make you successful (even if you "succeed") and so, by definition, it creates a life that isn't on your terms.

GETTING OUT OF YOUR OWN WAY

Our greatest frustration is not that we don't know what to do. It's that we know exactly what to do but we still don't do it.

– RICHARD WILKINS

I love this quote from my friend Richard Wilkins.

It sums up so much about the misunderstood challenges of most people's lives.

It sums up why simply learning more and more information, reading more and more books, taking more and more courses, seeing more and more therapists won't help you – why it *cannot* help you, because it's trying to fix the wrong problem. It's trying to fix a problem you don't have (knowing what to do), instead of the right problem (feeling safe to do it).

You don't need to learn anything.

You need to **unlearn** layers of limiting thinking patterns that work against your natural success and confidence mindset.

You need to **unlearn** layers of limiting thinking patterns that cause you to doubt and fear when your natural state is to simply move forward in a calm, methodical, workmanlike manner.

You need to **unlearn** layers of limiting thinking patterns that cause you to look for consequences instead of possibilities, to see lack instead of the abundance that is right in front of you.

To think small instead of relaxing into your unlimited potential.

To see yourself as unworthy and undeserving instead of as the incredible miracle you are.

Thinking patterns that tell you to fit in, play small, sacrifice your dreams and desires so as to not "show off."

To see taking care of yourself as being selfish.

To see pleasing others as more important than simply being and expressing all of who you are and setting free your incredible unique gifts for the benefit of the world.

All of this and much, much more you learned. But all of this is a web of lies. A toxic, awful, wicked and damaging belief matrix that is almost perfectly designed to block you from the success and confidence that is your birthright.

It isn't you, and the limits these thoughts create are false. <u>It is a prison without walls and without locks</u>.

You only need to be aware of the lies that you have been told and that you tell yourself in order to set yourself free.

And then not only will you know exactly what to do, **but you will actually do it**.

And then you can finally create a life that makes sense.

Now that you are free of the bad teaching and have your success mindset in place, this section of the book shows you two things: how to maintain your mind, because your mind is never static, and how to create the life of your dreams.

A FEW WORDS OF WARNING

Before we go further, I want to give you a few words of warning. Everything you've learned so far is exactly what you need to clear your mind of the bad programming and keep it clear.

But it only works if you maintain your mindset every day.

The good news is that your mind is not static. So, the way you think, the way you perceive the world, can be changed and shaped any way you want, provided you do that on purpose.

But equally and precisely, because your mind is not static, <u>you can fall back into the 99% ways of thinking</u>; the destructive thinking patterns that keep the 99% playing small.

By reading and then applying the knowledge in this book, you are well on your way to joining the 1%. But no one, and I mean **no one, gets permanent free membership**.

You only stay in the 1% club for as long as you keep your mind in tune with the 1% ways of thinking.

No one will check up on you; only you can do that for yourself. But if you don't maintain it, it will slowly fall away and all the incredible progress you've made, your new ways of thinking and living, will fall away with it.

As you go through this section, be careful not to lose sight of the thinking patterns and techniques from Step 2 – this is critical. You cannot create and maintain your new life without the right foundations in place. Trust me, I've made this mistake many times.

I remember both Stephen and Andy telling me that remaining conscious of the way I was thinking, of being aware when I started to fall back into old habits of thinking, was the key to creating the life that I wanted; that I needed to live thinking this way as a daily practice if I wanted this life.

It is a price that few chose to pay, but for those who do, the rewards are incredible.

MAINTAINING YOUR DEFAULT STATE

Your default state is the state you're most often in.

– JASON CAPITAL

This is why applying the knowledge within this book and rinsing and repeating until it becomes your default habit is so important. In the same way that you wash your body every day, so too, you need to clean your mind.

If you didn't wash every day, your body would get dirty, smelly, and likely diseased and infected.

Your mind is no different.

Working on my mindset is as much a part of my daily routine as getting up and having a shower, brushing my teeth, or having my morning coffee.

I have a daily routine that I simply do not compromise. I have learned through letting it slide too many times and seeing the consequences, that skipping or compromising on this routine results in my life being harder, more difficult, heavier, and my progress slower.

When I stick to this routine, my life is simply better. And, more importantly, it doesn't just stay better at the same level. It continues to improve.

The incredible news is that there is no limit to how well you can think. So, your progress, confidence, and success continue to accelerate.

The benefits from doing this each day never stop growing.

The whole purpose of my daily routine is to maintain my default state with this mindset.

Jason Capital has a great saying which is that "your default state is the state you're most often in." So each day, to reset and maintain your new mindset (your default), your routine should keep you in that state.

Soon enough the good habits will become as much of a reflex action as the bad habits were previously. This means that you win by default, on autopilot.

Each morning, the *very first thing I do* while I'm lying in bed for a few minutes before I get up is think about what I'm grateful for. Sometimes this is something simple and small like seeing the smile on my daughters' faces. Sometimes it's the sunrise. Sometimes I'm simply grateful for being alive and healthy, and for the day I'm about to live. Sometimes I'm grateful for the things that <u>didn't happen</u>, a reminder of how any fear is an illusion.

But no matter, I like to make sure that my very first thoughts are calm, grateful, and happy to ensure that my mind is tuned to seeing the abundance in my life as the very first thing it processes for the day, rather than any lack, resistance, or negativity.

I then get up and have my shower. While in the shower, I do focused daydreaming, where I am grateful for what is coming into my life. All the dreams and desires I am working on, I remain happy and grateful that they are coming my way.

Then once I'm up and dressed, I grab my coffee, sit at my desk, and spend a few minutes adding to my gratitude list (more on that later). This is a list of all the things that I have in my life, or that have happened – **or that haven't happened that I am grateful for.**

After spending a few minutes doing that, I take 5–10 minutes to first bring in the 15 seconds of positive thought and then some No Mind. Once I've done that, I feel calm, clearheaded, energized, and ready to deal with anything.

Throughout the day, I remain aware of how I'm feeling. I am looking for any bad feelings, any lack, any frustration, any negative thoughts. I scan my thoughts to see what tricks my ego is trying to use to bring me down, to keep me playing small.

I don't fight or resist it. I just accept completely that my ego will do this. Fighting it gives it power; observing it and becoming aware of its tricks takes away its power.

If I start feeling bad, I know it's time to slow down or stop, and bring in the 15 seconds of positive thought and No Mind. Then I'm reset. No matter what, three or four times per day, I will hold the 15 seconds and bring in No Mind.

To me it is now no different to getting a cup of coffee, to having a short break from work. It is simply a part of my normal routine. It just happens to be the single most powerful and effective part of that routine.

Finally, as I go to sleep at night, I spend a few minutes before I drift off bringing in No Mind. I remind myself all of the things I am grateful for and completely accept life as it is, knowing that whatever my life is, whatever has happened or is happening is exactly what I need to create my highest good. I let go of all fighting, judgement, and resistance and then drift off to sleep.

There is one more trick before you go to sleep that I will show you later on – just let me reveal that in the right time and right way for you.

By having this as my habit, as my daily routine, it means I am constantly making sure that the state I'm most often in is calm, grateful, unshakable, clear-minded, and at peace.

I always remember that my default state is the state I'm most often in.

It's hard to describe how good I feel when I do this. It's pretty hard to describe how much better my life has become since I've started living this way.

Is your ego telling you that what I've just described is really hard and sounds like a load of effort? That it sounds like hard work?

If so, well done for being aware of the latest trick your ego is pulling on you to keep you stuck – to get you to dismiss the answer that you've created in your life to create the life you want.

This isn't work – this is calm, peaceful, enjoyable. It is the very best way to relax and to create your dream life all at the same time. This is the most incredible way to give yourself a break and make yourself feel amazing all at once.

So don't let your ego derail you by trying to get you to associate this with hard work.

The key here is to recognize that all of the incredible benefits of thinking the right way only continue for as long as you continue to think the right way.

No longer being worried, scared, or anxious; no longer caught in the trap of negativity; no longer a prisoner to the awful toxicity of people pleasing; no longer bound by false limits.

Your ego will look to distract you away from doing the things that help you, the things that embed and enhance your thinking and pull you towards the things that erode it. One of the reasons I created my Instagram page was to create a system for me to stay tuned into this way of thinking every day.

NEW THINKING OFFERS NEW UNDERSTANDING

There's something really important I'd like you to consider now. "**When you change your thinking, you change your world.**" This is a great quote from Norman Vincent Peale and its power, when applied, is incredible.

And here's one example of how.

As you've gone through the chapters in the book so far, you've been changing your thinking. Your consciousness has been raising. And so, the way you see the world, yourself, and the possibilities for your life have been changing. Your mind has been opening as the thinking of the 99% and preconceived ideas have dissolved.

You have become a different person from the one you were when you first started reading this book.

What that means is that when you read any of the sections of this book a second time, you are able to understand more. In fact, you take in material that was always there but your previous level of consciousness had blocked you from seeing and understanding. Sections that you probably just skimmed over first time around suddenly hold incredible value and meaning for you.

Not because the material has changed but because you, your understanding, and your consciousness has changed.

This is true not just of this book but more broadly in your experiences in life. Each experience could only show you what your level of consciousness allowed you to access at the time. When you go back and look at those past experiences again, you can see things that were always there but were never visible to you until you changed your thinking.

Now this is where this gets even more powerful.

Consider that there is no limit to how well you can think, to how successful you can be, to how confident you can be.

There is no limit to how much you can grow and *be a better you*.

And that by being a better version of you, you can learn and apply more wisdom, feel better, and be more successful.

Each new (better) version of you allows you to access that knowledge at a deeper level; to see things; to understand things that you previously missed; to apply things and gain more wisdom from that application.

Don't just skip past that. Consider it for a while. See the virtuous circle of becoming more, which opens the door to more understanding and more possibilities, which, in turn, **allows you to become even more**.

And none of it is hard, or painful. It's fun and enjoyable as you unleash your natural success and confidence.

Can you see how the quality of your life reflects the quality of your thinking?

So now can you see how if you dip in and reread parts of this book, you will be able to access new wisdom and knowledge from the same material. Just doing a little bit each day adds up to big progress.

Can you also see why repetition is the master skill to unlocking wisdom?

Can you see how by skipping from one course to the next, from one book to the next, you don't gain the benefit that is waiting for you?

My strong counsel is that you read and reread the parts of this book that you feel you still need to master.

There is no rush here. The aim is to get the maximum benefit, not to rush on to the next book or course. If you slow down, you will see the truth in this.

RE-CONNECTING WITH YOUR SUPERPOWERS

Listen to your intuition. It will tell you everything you need to know.

– ANTHONY J. D'ANGELOU

One of the greatest gifts that comes from peeling away all the layers of damaging, muddled, and backwards thinking is that you start to reconnect again with your intuition and your subconscious mind.

These are your superpowers. We all have them – every single one of us, *including you*. It's just that most people don't know that they have them or doubt their power and so they limit their superpowers.

You start being free to think *what you really think*. And maybe for the first time since you were a child, you are free from the grip of the limiting and sabotaging thinking that captures 99% of the world.

More importantly, you can start to use your incredible mind to work for you on purpose instead of against you by accident.

You were born with a gift so powerful, so astonishing, that if you truly comprehended it, you would never, ever doubt yourself again. You have between your ears the most powerful supercomputer known to exist anywhere in the universe.

Its power is almost beyond comprehension, yet it goes largely unused by the vast majority of the world. It is astonishing in its <u>capacity</u>, breathtaking in its <u>adaptability</u>, awe-inspiring in its <u>ability to solve</u>

almost any problem. Its processing power is essentially unlimited.

Do you understand what that means?

You have been born with processing power in your head that is so powerful, science struggles to explain it.

Your subconscious mind processes (by the latest estimates) more than 40 million bits of information per second.

Just to put this in context, in 2014 the world's fastest supercomputer at the time, the K Supercomputer in Okinawa, Japan, *took 40 minutes to simulate a single second of human brain activity.*

Your subconscious mind on autopilot uses that incredible power to process partial, incomplete, and often downright inaccurate information to give you insights, ideas, and breakthroughs that logically seem impossible.

But because 99% of people's minds are filled with bad programming, they don't and can't use this incredible power to create the lives they dream of.

Your ego right now will still be desperate for you to be one of them. It will tell you that you're not special because everyone has this power. It will tell you that it isn't much use having a superpower if you're not yet living the life that you want. It will tell you that I can't be right about this, otherwise you would have had more success by now.

But that's only because you haven't been able to access that power, not because it isn't there.

But now, as you've peeled away the layers and layers of bad programming, your intuition – your superpower – is yours to access once again.

It is the opposite of your ego. It is the little genius inside you, waiting to serve you and to help you fulfill the dreams and desires that sit within you. It is your very best friend who you can 100% rely on, provided you work with it, instead of ignoring it.

I literally instruct my subconscious mind to give me answers every day. And it never, ever fails me.

This is a trick that Thomas Edison used and it is astonishing in its power. Edison said: "Never go to sleep without a request to your subconscious."

This is problem solving the easy (natural) way and it is the gift your subconscious mind and your intuition gives you.

Before you go to sleep, tell your subconscious mind the problem you need an answer to, the problem you've previously struggled to solve and need a solution for.

Then go to sleep, **_knowing 100% that your subconscious mind will give you the answers you need_**.

I have instructed my subconscious mind to give me answers to business issues, personal challenges, financial questions, and problems where I had absolutely no idea what possible solution there could be.

I simply instructed my subconscious mind to provide me with a solution to problem X and went to sleep.

Sometimes I would wake up and immediately get the answer I needed. Sometimes the answer came later. But it will happen. What you'll find is that the next day or in the following days, during some mundane activity like taking a shower, brushing your teeth, going for a walk, or making a coffee, an answer will just pop into your mind.

When it arrives, the answer will seem so incredibly obvious you'll wonder why you hadn't already thought of it. It will give you exactly what you need to answer the question, resolve the issue, or deal with the challenge that you're facing.

Just as powerfully, by stilling your mind, being in control of your thoughts, and being free of all the bad programming, you tune into your intuition in everything that you deal with. What that means is that you'll be closely attuned to what your intuition is saying about the decision you should make, the people you should speak to, the small and seemingly insignificant actions you should take, or the thing you should do next, even if doesn't consciously make sense.

I have found, on countless occasions, that I simply had a strong feeling to do something – to contact a particular person, to say yes or no to a specific opportunity or deal – and that what's emerged afterwards has shown just how right that decision was.

It is <u>staggering</u> the pain I have avoided, the bad decisions I have averted, the money I haven't wasted, the time I have saved, the incredible opportunities I have found, the astonishing people I have met, all from following my intuition.

I have lost count of the number of times people have asked me how I "knew" something was the right answer. And it was simply that my mind was clear of bad programming; I was in control of my thoughts and I was therefore conscious and attuned to my intuition.

My subconscious mind had already pieced everything together even if I couldn't explain how. The incredible power of my subconscious mind (just like the incredible power of yours) was there to give me exactly <u>what I needed</u>, exactly <u>when I needed it</u>. It had worked through all of the partial, incomplete data and come up with an incredible, perfect answer.

This superpower is now yours too, if you've followed the steps outlined in the earlier sections of this book.

THINKING FOR YOURSELF AGAIN

When you find yourself on the side of the majority,
it's time to pause and reflect.

– MARK TWAIN

You are now free to think for yourself, to consciously think your own thoughts instead of unconsciously thinking the thoughts of the masses.

But will you use this power?

Consider: How often you have gone against what the majority thinks or says? Consider the clothes you wear, the way you live your life, the social, moral, political, religious, or spiritual beliefs you have, how you spend your time. How different has this been for you from the majority of the people around you?

That doesn't mean these choices are wrong; it means they have been choices made without really thinking about them. Most people fall into lazy, herd mentality habits of thinking – <u>which is really another way of saying that they stop thinking for themselves</u>.

And as a result, you become detached from your own thinking, from your own values and priorities, and you start letting others think for you. It's how you start to veer off your own path, your true path, and start walking along the well-trodden path others would choose for you.

In a world of social media and the false urgency and drama of the 24-hour news cycle, it's easy to fall into herd thinking. You stop being connected to your subconscious mind and your intuition about what is right, what makes sense, and what works for you in any situation. **You block your superpowers**.

Giving power and control over your thoughts consciously or unconsciously means you stop looking at things with your own eyes, your own mind, and just accepting the opinion of others, the opinions of the masses, as "the way things should be."

Your mind closes to everything except the possibilities, options, and opportunities the herd wants you to see. And your world grows poorer and smaller as a result.

By remembering to consider if you are the controller of your thoughts, you give yourself the freedom to look at everything without preconceptions.

By being the controller of your thoughts, instead of falling into lazy, herd thinking, you can remain open-minded and look for what's really true and, more importantly, what's true, right, or what makes sense <u>for you</u>.

And it is only by truly thinking for yourself that you <u>start acting for yourself</u>. Only then can you start creating a life that makes sense for you.

And that's what we're going to do next.

THINGS TO CONSIDER

- Can you now see the real possibilities for your life? Possibilities that were always there but simply hidden from you in plain sight, by the sabotaging, negative programming you had been given?

- Can you now see the person you are capable of becoming? Once you learn to control your mind, the possibility of becoming that person turns into a probability.

- Can you see how confidence, success, achievement, wealth, and happiness is simply a process?

- Can you see that without making controlling your mind a way of life, you will fall back into the thinking of the 99%?

- Consider that your default state is the state you are most often in. Consider the possibilities for your life from understanding the power of this statement.

- Consider how the possibilities for your life never stop expanding once you start thinking in the right ways.

- Consider how your understanding, your ability to access the benefits of this material and all material you read, becomes greater the more you elevate your thinking.

CHAPTER 12

THE INCREDIBLE POWER
OF AUTHENTICITY: PART 1

**The privilege of a lifetime is to become
who you truly are.**

CARL JUNG

L et me ask you a question.

When was the last time you were really you?

When you spoke freely, acted freely, lived freely? When you weren't thinking about what you should be, should do, and should think?

When was the last time you were 100%, fully, unapologetically you, <u>without holding anything back</u>?

The honest answer for most is "a long time ago," probably when you were just a young child; when you hadn't yet taken on board all the rules, all the "shoulds," the false blueprints for who you were supposed to be and the life you were supposed to live.

Think about that for a second. Nearly everyone you meet, nearly everyone you interact with, isn't being the real, fully authentic version of themselves. They are all, in some way, pretending or trying to be something other than who they really are in order to fit in with the constraints of society and be accepted by those around them.

The process of being "socialized" is one that makes you less real, less authentic, and makes you live less honestly as you're taught to bend yourself out of shape, pretend to be something you're not, and hide the parts of you that don't align with the model that society says we should all adopt.

The world is filled with people trying to be something different from who they really are, unconsciously trying to be *inauthentic*. And then we wonder why there are such widespread issues of depression, anxiety, and mental health.

It shouldn't be a surprise to anyone that pushing people to fit into a preset mold – and punishing them if they don't – is a recipe for failure, misery, and a lack of confidence for the majority of people.

They (like you) were constantly told that they were not good enough, not right, getting it wrong, were failing, and so on, <u>for simply being who they are</u>.

When you were a young child, you were naturally confident and successful and you were **fully authentic**. You achieved more incredible things in those first few years of your life than at any other time.

You expressed exactly what you thought and felt, you wore the clothes you wanted to, you chose the toys you wanted to play with, you knew exactly what you wanted, and you reacted badly when someone tried to get you to do something you didn't like, didn't want, or that didn't make sense to you.

All the shoulds weren't yet barriers to you being who you really were and creating the life you wanted to live.

That was you in your natural state – naturally confident, naturally successful, completely authentic.

You weren't <u>trying</u> to be confident or successful then. You just were. Because you hadn't yet learned that you were supposed to be anything other than who you were.

Over time you were taught all the rules, all the "shoulds" that your parents, teachers, friends, and wider society pushed into you. You learned it so well that like most people you stopped even realizing that there were rules, and it just became the unconscious "truth," the unquestioned way life "should be." You stopped considering; you stopped questioning; you stopped fighting against it.

You became programmed.

But the problem is that <u>those rules weren't your rules</u>. Those "shoulds" weren't your "shoulds." That blueprint for life wasn't your blueprint even though you came to think it was.

It became "who you are" but at some deep level it felt wrong, incongruous, and uncomfortable. You stopped liking the person you became with all the suffocating, stifling rules and "shoulds" that made you miserable and squashed your dreams and desires.

And then others told you (or you told yourself) the lie that you "lacked confidence," another way in which you were "not measuring up" against a false standard.

Can you see the insanity of this process?

You are told to be something you're not; to think in ways that don't make sense you; to act in ways that don't reflect who you are or who you want to be; to make choices that don't work for you and don't align with your authentic desires.

And you are punished for breaking these rules. You are made to strive after a false standard that takes you into misery, not into happiness and success.

And then you are "treated" for the very misery, unhappiness, and lack of self-esteem and success that this process **inevitably** creates. It is dangerous, nasty, wicked, toxic insanity.

But the truth is that there's nothing wrong with you, **_the real you_**. It's not the real you that you don't like and don't feel confident about. It's the _false you_, measured against the false standards that others gave you.

When you realize the truth that it's not the real you but your ego (your false self) that you don't like, then the whole equation of confidence and self-doubt transforms.

You understand that the real you is separate from the toxic programming that nearly everyone has been programmed with. It sets you free to respect, like, and love yourself again.

To just be you again.

That is natural confidence and, in this chapter, now that you've cleaned away the bad programming and started to see the real you again, we're going to go through the process of once again becoming completely, authentically you.

And as a result, you'll be going through the process of becoming the person you want to be, instead of the person that you "should" be. Then, and only then, can you begin creating the life you dream of and a life that makes sense to you.

CREATING THE RIGHT BLUEPRINT FOR YOUR LIFE

You'll learn, as you get older, that rules are made to be broken. Be bold enough to live life on your terms, and never, ever apologize for it. Go against the grain, refuse to conform, take the road less travelled instead of the well-beaten path. And stubbornly refuse to fit in.

– MANDY HALE

One of the most important things I worked through with my coach and mentor Stephen as I was going through my divorce was designing a new blueprint for my life. This wasn't about what I wanted to have in my life – things like my perfect partner, finding my purpose, creating the wealth I desired and so on. That would come later (and I will show you how in a later chapter in this book).

This was instead creating a new blueprint, a new set of rules. These were my authentic rules: my way to live and *my way* to navigate through *my life*. These were rules and a blueprint that would help me become and to live as the very best version of me.

Stephen showed me that to achieve my dreams, I had to become the best version of me, because it was the very best version of the real, authentic me who would make those dreams a reality.

I had to become the person I wanted to be <u>in order to create</u> the life I wanted to live.

By understanding, probably for the first time since I was a child, who I was and what the very best version of me looked like, my efforts could start focusing on living in ways that <u>helped</u> me instead of <u>harmed</u> me; ways that accelerated my progress, confidence, happiness, and growth instead of blocking them. My focus would set me free to be all of who I was and all of who I could be instead of keeping me a prisoner.

And that same focus would unleash my true potential which would otherwise stay bottled up, frustrated, and worthless as I worked to be something I wasn't; to build a life that wasn't my own and a life that wouldn't and couldn't make me happy.

Confidence, happiness, and success comes from who you are, not from what you have.

It's completely normal and natural to want the very best that life has to offer: health, wealth, love, respect, sex, and material abundance. But your happiness and success cannot and does not come from external "stuff"; otherwise, if the stuff goes, so does your confidence.

This means it never really existed in the first place.

We are taught to think that when we get the stuff, we will be happy and confident and feel successful. But success is a process, which means doing the right things in the right order. And the right order is that you have to be happy and confident with who you are first, you have to get your mind right first, and then all the stuff naturally follows after that.

The right blueprint for your life has three parts.

The first and most important is about getting clear about what the <u>very best version of you looks like</u>. This is the real you, but, more importantly, the very best you.

The second part is defining <u>the new set of rules</u> for how you live your life. The previous section of this book was about making you aware of all the bad rules that most people live by that keep them small, destroy their confidence, and crush their dreams. This second part is about designing a new set of rules that help you live authentically and so your best life.

The last part (which I cover in a later chapter) is about <u>getting clear on what you want</u>. But you can only really know what you truly want when you know who you truly are. That's why it was so important to peel back the bad programming first and to get you to fully reconnect with who you really are before you start looking at what you want; otherwise, the danger is that you start going after the wrong things.

BECOMING THE VERY BEST YOU

I am. Two of the most powerful words, for what you put after them shapes your reality.

– BEVAN LEE

One of the biggest hidden blocks to feeling good about who you are and being who you want to be is the labels we allow ourselves to be given.

As you grow up, you get told by your parents, siblings, teachers, and friends what type of person "you are." You get told that you are happy, bossy, charming, grumpy, shy, depressed, clever, fat, sporty, and hundreds more labels just like them.

And equally you get told about the kinds of things that "someone like you" can or cannot be, do, or have.

Over time you consciously or unconsciously start to accept these labels as facts. They become your identity. And this identity profoundly shapes your experience of life and your experience of who you are.

You take on the behaviors that flow from that identity.

The possibilities and limits you define for yourself stem from those labels. The feelings and experiences you believe are available to you follow from that definition.

Without realizing it, you shut down and put away big parts of who you are in order to align with this identity – an identify that is made up of a bunch of labels that you were casually and arbitrarily given.

So consider for a moment, what labels were you given?

Do these labels help you or harm you on your journey to being who you want to be?

You can cast off these labels any time you choose, because they are opinions not facts. You can pick any new labels you like.

Consider for a moment who you could be and what you could do if you dropped the labels that hurt you and only moved forward with ones that helped you.

That is what we're doing now. You are giving yourself the freedom to define who you are, in alignment with your own labels.

Remember as you go through this section that this is about you becoming the very best version of yourself – becoming all you can be. It's not about becoming someone you're not. It's about unlocking everything within you.

Your ego will want to turn this into you somehow feeling bad or inadequate because you are not that person right now. That is a trick and a trap to keep you stuck and playing small.

Be excited about this, because you're now moving quickly towards becoming that incredible, astonishing, and amazing version of you – the version that has always been there. This is you being repatterned to be

<u>who you were meant to be</u>.

I loved this process; it was one of the most enjoyable things I've ever done.

Through it, I learned how I had allowed others to define who I was and who I could be – as well as what my possibilities and limitations were. But more importantly, I learned how little truth there were in the labels I had been given; how I had lived up to this small version of myself because I thought that was who I was.

This was the exact process I went through with Stephen to reconnect with the real me. **Remember, the real you is the person you dream of being**. The person you've lived your life as so far is your ego-driven self.

Before we start, take a moment to ensure you are in control of your thoughts, to ensure you are conscious enough to see clearly what you really want and what others expect of you. This is about you designing you and being authentic – the expectations of others have no part to play in that at all.

Take out a piece of paper. Then close your eyes and allow yourself to daydream about the very best, the ultimate, the greatest version of you.

See you in your mind. See what you look like having become that incredible, astonishing person. See your energy, your confidence, your natural calmness and authority, your unshakableness.

See how you dress; see your posture; feel the feelings you feel as this person. See the certainty; the trust you feel in yourself; the complete sense that no matter what, you are, and will be, just fine.

Really immerse yourself; soak yourself in this vision, in these feelings. Explore every aspect of you that you desire to explore, every facet of how you think, feel, act, and behave; the feelings you have; how you deal with situations. See how you speak, the tone and cadence of your voice. See the calm energy with which you look at and interact with people. See how unhurried you are; how in command of your life you are.

See how fearless you are; how kind you are; how authentic and natural you are.

When you're ready, open your eyes and write down in detail that vision of that very best version of you.

You can do this as a mind map, as a list, or just as a description. Write down all the qualities, all the facets, all the talents unleashed, all the feelings, the energy you feel as this person. See the behaviors you now have. Write it all down.

Don't place any limits on yourself. Any time you hear that voice in your head say "you can't do that" or "that's not realistic," "that's never going to happen," "stop being silly," or anything that causes you to hold back on this, that's your ego talking. It is trying to keep you thinking in the same ways as you have in the past, to keep you stuck, and to keep you from living the life you want.

Any limits are your ego's way of sabotaging you. Each time you feel like you want to put something down, do it, no matter how much that voice tells you it's wrong or stupid to do.

The more detail you put down for this, the more it will help you. If you feel stuck, one trick is to literally just started writing. Write down the very first thing that you see or feel about that vision of yourself in your mind. Don't focus on getting the words perfect; you can always refine this later. For now, capture the feelings.

There is only one rule for how you write this down.

I will explain this rule in more detail slightly later in the book, but for now, as you write this down, write it as a description of the person **that you have already become**. It should be in the *past tense* as you look back on who you have already become. Don't write it in the present tense, and definitely not in the future tense (i.e., as the person you one day hope to be).

This needs to be in the past tense – *something that has already happened*. I want you to describe the person that you've already become.

This is the process for designing the real you – the best you – that will inevitably create the life you desire to live. It is this person who is the real you when all the bullshit layers of bad programming, stifling social conditioning, and terrible teaching are peeled away.

This is the person you were designed to become, the person you are destined to be, and the person that every experience, every challenge, every difficulty is building you towards.

Here's why this process matters.

This is the real you. You simply haven't been living as that person because you haven't realized it's the real you. Now you have that choice.

How you express that choice is that in any situation, you choose to live yourself in alignment with your design of you, in alignment with the choices that the best version of you would make.

Your job now is to, in a calm workmanlike way, live in alignment with that design instead of accidently living in alignment with the limited version of you, weighed down by all the bad programming.

Let me give you an example.

When I did my design of me, one of the most important qualities in my design was being completely in control of my mind, completely calm, serene, and unshakable no matter what.

So, in every meeting at work, on every date I went on, when anything frustrating, annoying, or difficult happened, I reminded myself that I was unshakable; that this was who I really was and that it was only my ego and bullshit programming that blocked me from experiencing that.

Each situation became a checkpoint, a reminder for how much I was living as the real me. I came to really look forward to any situation that could challenge my calmness, my unshakableness. It was my chance to live the real me at a new and higher level. It was a check as to whether I was living authentically as the best me or whether I was living small, allowing the unhelpful programming to get in my way.

I never felt bad if I realized that I was playing small. Instead, I was really pleased with myself *for noticing that I was*. This meant I was aware of what was happening; I was back in control and able to change straightaway. This was a choice that 99% of people are never even conscious of.

And each time I became aware that I was not living in alignment with my design was another step closer to me becoming that person.

Awareness was how the battle was won.

Soon enough, unshakable became my default. Soon enough, the best version of me (the one that I designed) became my default setting instead of the programmed version of me.

Your ego will want you to see this as a switch being flicked, to see this change in binary terms. Be aware that this is a trap.

It wants you to use each occasion where you are not living as the best version of you as a stick to beat you with, as something to make you feel bad.

Your ego will look to use any "slip up," any moment when you didn't do this "perfectly" as a way to tell you that you've failed; that this isn't working and that you should just give up and go back to your old habits of thinking.

What your ego won't show you the incredible benefits of living in alignment with your design **for some of the time instead of none of the time**. It will present you with this bullshit binary view that you either do it perfectly 100% of the time or that you've failed.

When that thought comes up, just consider the benefits of living as the best you <u>more of the time</u>.

Success and confidence are achieved by realizing the incredible truth of who you are and in a calm workmanlike way changing your default setting back to your naturally confident and successful state. It took many years to program you out of this natural way of thinking. Don't expect it to reverse instantly.

But...

When you follow the process I've described, you and your life can change very quickly. And you can change your default setting most of the time. I found that within a few weeks of designing the best me I was living in alignment with that design about 55% of the time. Within a few months, I had got that to about 80% of the time, and after a year to about 90%.

Can you imagine how great you would feel to be living as the real you 55% of the time (i.e., the majority of your time) within a few weeks? Can you imagine how much more progress you would make, how great you would feel, how much more confident you would be living as the very best version of you within a few weeks?

So, beware your ego telling you that you're a little bit crap every time you get something wrong instead of seeing the truth of all the incredible progress you can and will make in a few weeks, if you choose to.

Remember, one thought helps you and the other harms you. The trick of life is choosing the thoughts that help you.

CREATING THE NEW RULES

The second part of the blueprint for an authentic, confident, and successful life is to create the rules for you to live by. Think of this as your code for life. It is the set of rules you *consciously* choose to govern your life.

Almost everyone has a set of rules like this, but in the overwhelming majority of cases these rules have been chosen unconsciously and are simply the inherited jumble of things you've been told you "should."

Have you ever stopped to consider the rules you live by before? To consider whether the rules that govern your life are the ones you would consciously choose?

When you were first born you didn't have any rules to live by. You were taught a set of rules directly and indirectly by your family, friends, teachers, and wider society – rules that you "must" follow in order to fit in.

The problem is that so many of these rules are just the "way things are done" rather than being there to help you.

Consider for a moment: <u>Is there any benefit in following a rule that doesn't help you</u>? Is there any benefit in you not considering and not consciously choosing the rules that you follow?

We spend the first part of children's lives putting them in a confined box of rules and social conditioning, teaching them blind obedience (note the word "blind," as in, without questioning, without seeing, without thinking). They are taught to follow rules whether or not they work for them, help them, or harm them.

Then later in life, people spend huge amounts of time, money, and effort trying to "fix" themselves through personal development and therapy; to overcome the very misery created by the terrible rules that they were institutionalized with in the first place.

Here's the truth:

Any rule only has value if it helps you, those you love, and the wider world. Ideally it should do all three.

Most rules that most people follow do none of those three things.

And conforming and fitting in isn't a benefit, despite what others may tell you. It is simply a form of control.

So, the rules *that you choose for you* need to be chosen with great care. Despite what most of the world thinks, the purpose of the rules for your life is to <u>expand your life</u>, happiness, joy, confidence, and success – <u>not to limit them</u>. They exist to set you free, not to place limits on you.

This is the reverse of almost everyone's experience of rules, which have mainly been about stopping, limiting, or preventing you from doing, thinking, being, or acting in particular ways. Those are the rules that are created to control others. *They exist to make you serve others rather than to serve and support yourself.*

What we are defining here are the rules that *will set you free* to be fully authentic and to have you live your life on your terms. *This is about how you take charge of your life.*

Remember, confident and successful people, the 1%, establish their own rules, consciously, purposefully, and deliberately. And there is only one question they ask to decide if they are worthwhile: *Do they work?*

So take a moment to consider the rules that would set you free to be fully you; the rules that would lead you to living life 100% on your terms. I went through this exact process with my coach Stephen and I keep my rules on my phone and I take them with me wherever I go. Whenever I am facing any situation, I remind myself of my rules for my life.

They are my guide to decide what I should do, alongside my values. I review them regularly to make sure that they are indeed helping me live my best, most authentic life. I am in control of them, which means I *can change them any time I like*, but only in such a way that helps me live my best life, never to play small and shrink backwards from life.

As you come up with your rules, keep in mind that vision of the greatest version of yourself, the real you. What are the rules that the best version of you would have?

To help you, I've listed out some of my rules below. Feel free to use them exactly, to change them, to come up with new ones, or to come up with completely different ones. This is just for you.

1. I don't accept others rules – I define my own.

2. I make the intelligent but bold choice to not play small, ever.

3. I am 100% authentically me, no matter what.

4. I say "no" to things that don't work for me and that don't align with my values.

5. I spend time every day working on my mind.

6. I am clear and direct in my communication.

7. I am kind, decent, and act with integrity but I will never tolerate anything less than the same from other people in my life.

8. No negativity.

9. I do not let anyone treat me badly, ever, under any circumstances.

10. I ask for what I want and express how I feel.

11. I put myself first, because only then can I give the very best of myself to others.

12. I am 100% responsible for the quality of my life.

13. I observe, not judge.

14. I look for and take the benefits from every situation and leave the baggage behind.

15. I remember that everything works out for the best.

16. I don't hide any part of me away or pretend to be something I'm not.

17. I don't seek anyone's approval, ever.

18. I accept that the only thing I can control is my mind. I work diligently on achieving the outcomes I desire but I detach from needing any specific outcome to happen.

19. I live in alignment with the truth that failure is how success is achieved.

20. My job is to be the very best version of me, always. I recognize and completely accept that some people will love me, and some will not, and I am completely OK with both. My measure is how I feel about me.

21. I recognize that fear is an illusion my ego uses to keep me playing small. So I never allow my fears to limit my choices.

22. My highest goal is my happiness.

23. Fuck being realistic.

24. I focus on progress not perfection; momentum is my friend.

Take some time to come up with your own list of rules. There can be as many or as few you as makes sense to you.

The point of writing them down is so that you become conscious of them – so you go and LIVE THEM.

Remember, **unapplied knowledge has no value at all**. The value comes from the application. As you apply these rules, as you try them on for size, you will see what works for you and what doesn't; what rules need to change and what new rules need to be added.

Each day you live in alignment with these rules is a day you take a <u>massive step</u> towards being that greatest version of yourself and towards creating the life that you desire. It is how you live life on your terms and live as part of the 1%.

AUTHENTICITY AND INTEGRITY ARE TWO SIDES OF THE SAME COIN

Honesty is more than not lying. It is truth telling, truth speaking, truth living, and truth loving.

– JAMES E. FAUST

One of the most crucial aspects of living authentically is to act with complete integrity.

Integrity is the practice of not only being honest but of showing a consistent and uncompromising adherence to your principles; in your case, this means your values and your rules.

It means not lying to others, and, more importantly, not lying to yourself. It means staying true to yourself (your values and your rules) no matter the situation or circumstance. To not stay true to yourself means the greatest sacrifice of all: the sacrifice of you being who you really are.

If you watch any courtroom, the oath each witness must give is that they will "tell the truth, the whole truth, and nothing but the truth." Imagine if you made that same vow to yourself.

That you would live truthfully, fully and completely truthfully, in every aspect of your life. And that you would only live truthfully, with nothing shaded, no messages "managed," spun, or massaged; no inconvenient bits hidden.

Living the life you want to live and becoming the person you want to be only happens when you refuse to compromise your integrity and values.

When what you say, what you think, and what you do all line up.

Integrity and authenticity are what I call "meta-values," by which I mean they are the foundation stone for all other values.

Integrity is authentic behavior that requires no permission or acknowledgement from anyone else.

Integrity means speaking your mind, going for what you want and what you think is right, and being unafraid of others' opinions.

It means showing up as the same person at home, with your friends, at work, or with your partner. You don't shade who you are or what you think to suit the occasion or audience.

It means not bitching about your partner to your friends and then about your friends to your partner.

It means you are up front and honest with people.

Most people like to think they have integrity, but the truth is their integrity and good intentions are overridden by an addiction to people pleasing.

So their fear of upsetting others, of going against the grain, of saying truthful but unpopular things causes them to lose their integrity. They carry their childlike habits with them into adulthood. They are afraid of getting "into trouble" if they speak their mind, go against the grain, or break the rules.

And in doing so, they betray their authentic selves, because they are focused on what they "should" think, say, or do rather than what they really think, or want to say or do.

You may lose some "friends" when you live this way, but realize that most people choose to lose themselves instead.

Consider which is really the greatest loss.

What you gain, though, is the complete freedom and indestructible self-respect that can only come from a refusal to live life on other's terms.

Freedom from the need to constantly trying to figure out what you "should' think, say, or do; freedom from having to be a chameleon and always having to blend in.

WHY THE TRUTH WILL SET YOU FREE

If you ask people whether they would prefer the difficult truth or comfortable lies, almost universally people will say that they want the truth.

But look at their actions and you will see that they really prefer comfortable lies.

They avoid saying what they really think, what they really feel, or what they really want for fear of upsetting others or creating an uncomfortable, confrontational situation.

So they shade the truth, spin it, soften it, "manage the message."

Equally, most people only like to listen to the "truths" they want to hear and get affronted when something jars with their sense of how the world should be.

The problem with not being <u>fully honest</u> with yourself and others is that it doesn't help anyone.

When you lie to someone (and that includes yourself), you are communicating that you don't think they (you) <u>can handle the truth</u>.

That is disrespectful and patronizing.

You cannot feel good about yourself or others in a matrix of lies, however well-intentioned those lies may be. And what if those lies are the very things that are keeping them (or you) trapped, unhappy, and playing small?

What if the truth would quite literally set them (or you) free to be all that you wanted to be and live the life you wanted to live? A true friend, a person of integrity, does the right thing even when it's hard – especially when it hard, in fact, because that's when it matters the most.

The 1% who get to live life on their terms don't fear – indeed, they actively embrace – the truth in all aspects of their lives. They only want to give and receive the truth because they know it is a precious gift that holds incredible value.

They know the consequences of lies and misguided best intentions are vastly more damaging than any truth could ever be. Say your truth with kindness and respect, but do say it. It's a gift that very few people give.

THINGS TO CONSIDER

- Consider: When was the last time you were really you?

- Whose rules, whose blueprint for your life are you following? Did you consciously choose these rules or have you unconsciously accepted the rules that others said you should follow?

- What labels have you been given that you no longer need? What new labels could you now choose that help you?

- Consider if the person that you dream of being is the person that you really are; that the only thing that is blocking you from being that person right now is your ego. Don't rush past this point. Slow down and consider what this means for your life.

- Be aware of your ego telling you that you either live this new way perfectly, 100% of the time, or that you've "failed." Ask yourself if this way of thinking helps you or harms you.

- Consider the benefits to you and your life of living this way more of the time.

- What rules will **you** now choose for **your life**?

- Consider the freedom of never again having to pretend to be someone or something that you're not. Consider the freedom to be 100% you.

CHAPTER 13

THE INCREDIBLE POWER OF AUTHENTICITY: PART 2

We ask ourselves, "Who am I to be brilliant, gorgeous, talented, and fabulous?" Actually, who are you not to be? Your playing small does not serve the world. There is nothing enlightened about shrinking so that other people will not feel insecure around you. As we let our own light shine, we unconsciously give other people permission to do the same. As we are liberated from our own fear, our presence automatically liberates others.

MARIANNE WILLIAMSON

Authenticity is the opposite of people pleasing. It is the antidote to people pleasing. It means being authentic even when, *most importantly when*, others disapprove of who you are.

And so often that disapproval comes when you seek to unleash your best self, your talents, and your gifts.

In one of my sessions with Stephen, we were discussing how to be authentic in the different environments and contexts that we all face in our daily lives. I made a comment (the importance of which I completely missed initially) where I talked about adapting who I was depending on the situation I was facing; how I had hidden my talents away, talents I knew I had, so that I would be accepted and would fit in.

Stephen didn't initially respond and instead just calmly smiled and looked at me to see if I had noticed what I had just said.

After one of the pauses that were his signal to me to take a moment to consider what I had just said, he simply said, "False modesty is still false. Do you like lying to yourself? Do you like playing small?"

He was not suggesting that I spend my time walking around and bragging. He was simply asking me why I felt the need to be dishonest with myself about who I was, about the talents that I had, and about the gifts that I had been given.

The choice was not to brag or not brag; that was my ego talking.

The real choice was to live in full expression of my talents – calmly, kindly, and with a view to being of service to the world – or to play small, to let those talents remain hidden away and, in effect, useless.

He was showing me that I had fallen into the trap of playing small in order to not upset others and in doing so I was limiting my life; I was limiting the possibilities for what I could achieve and who I could become.

I had allowed my ego to confuse something good (not being conceited and bragging) with something bad (lying and pretending I was something less than I really was). And as a result, I would not and could not unleash the greatness within me.

And the same is true for you.

Whatever you focus on expands, so when you focus on playing small so as not to upset, intimidate, or offend others, you find more and more reasons to play small – until playing small is what you do by default.

Have you fallen into this trap?

Do you hide yourself away because of concern over the reaction of others?

Do you put away your talents? Do you dim your shine? Do you allow yourself to be less than you are in order to make others feel in some way better?

We are taught the toxic, wicked belief that letting your light shine, that giving full reign to your talents and gifts is "showing off." This is horrible, nasty, deceitful teaching that causes untold damage.

It is wrong, wrong, wrong.

Consider for a moment how insane this way of thinking is; and yet, most of the world accepts it unconsciously.

You are expected and you allow yourself to become much less, to do much less, to live much less, to enjoy much less, to have much less happiness in order to avoid the risk that someone else "might" not want you to be all of who you are.

So each interaction causes more and more people to become and have less.

And so pretty soon, 99% of the world lives to a tiny fraction of their potential because of a fear that someone might not <u>like you being all of who you are</u> – despite the fact that the world <u>needs you to be all of who you are</u>.

To unleash your talents and gifts in the service of those around you; to give and contribute to your highest level, not to your lowest; to give the world your best, not some half-baked, stunted version.

Imagine what the world would be like if 99% of people lived to their highest potential and lifted those around them to do the same. Imagine how many problems would simply cease to exist. Imagine if you stepped outside of this stifling thought pattern and set those around you free.

Isn't that worth the risk of intimidating or upsetting someone who would prefer that you played small?

SEEING YOUR TALENTS AS CLEARLY AS YOUR FAULTS

How easily do you see and accept the good in yourself?

Can you look at who you are, what you've done, the way you look, the decisions you've made, the things you've achieved, etc., and see the good, the really good, and the absolutely amazing?

The vast majority's default lens on themselves and on their life is on the negative – not just seeking but actively *amplifying* anything they perceive as less than perfect about themselves.

And then they present this as the truth and broadcast it to themselves 24/7/365. But this isn't your natural way to think. Just consider if this had been your natural way to think, do you think as a species it would have helped us survive, grow, and evolve?

From an early age, most people get taught that loving yourself is arrogance and conceit and that you should instead be humble. And most people are taught that their value comes from what they do, not who they are.

And so, because you learn (erroneously) that you don't have *inherent* value but only *functional* value (for your talents, your looks, the money you bring in, the chores you do, the service you provide to others, etc.), you learn to start comparing your value with others.

And because standard schooling and most parenting focuses on what you've got wrong and what you need to get better at, you learn again and again to seek out your shortcomings, instead of your gifts; to focus on where you are less than others and need to "improve" rather than to understand all the ways in which you are amazing, wonderful, talented, and uniquely gifted.

Imagine, instead, if the default approach was to identify and amplify all your natural gifts. Imagine if you were taught, parented, socialized that you were precious, wonderful, incredible for being, not simply for doing or having?

This is one of the reasons I have no time for the "fake it till you make it" approach to success that so many people advocate. You don't need to fake anything.

When you look to fake a behavior, a feeling, or an identity, you are pretending. You're being fake and you know that you're faking it.

It's way, way, way, way better to simply realize the truth: that the most empowering thought is also the most truthful and accurate; that you are enough; that you are talented beyond measure; that you have incredible gifts.

All you need to do is set them free. Those aren't fake gifts, pretend gifts, things you're making up. They are as real as the chair you're sitting in.

You have no need to fake anything. Simply being you, fully, unapologetically, with love and respect, is the most powerful, life-changing, confidence-affirming, success-creating thing you can do.

Then, instead of you bending yourself out of shape, to live dishonestly to fit in with the world, you can live honestly and the world will adjust to fit in with you.

RESETTING YOUR RELATIONSHIP WITH YOURSELF

Putting yourself first doesn't mean you don't care about others. It means you're smart enough to know that you cannot help others if you don't help yourself first.

– ANONYMOUS

How would you rate your relationship with yourself?

If you were to score your relationship with yourself out of 10, what score would you give it? Answer honestly, as this is only for your benefit. Look to how you feel rather than how you think, as it is your feelings that show the truth.

Here's why this matters.

The quality of your relationship with yourself **defines your ability to actually be yourself**.

The more you respect, like, cherish, and love yourself the more you will actually be who you really are. The less you like yourself, the less you respect and love yourself, the more you feel like you should pretend to be someone and something other than who you authentically are.

So, let me ask you a different question: **Do you love yourself?**

Do you love who you are? Do you feel excited about being you? Would you be comfortable telling people that you love yourself? Would you feel proud to tell the world that you genuinely and deeply love you, in the same way that you would feel proud to say that you love your partner, your family, your children, your pets?

If not, have you stopped to consider **why not**?

We are taught that completely and unconditionally loving another is wonderful, something to aspire to, almost the pinnacle of the human experience.

Yet, we are also taught that feeling the same way about ourselves is somehow bad; that loving yourself is somehow vain, arrogant, conceited, and even narcissistic.

And so most people are desperately uncomfortable with giving themselves love because of a false fear – because of a lie that this most natural and human of feelings, to simply love who you really are, is terrible and conceited.

It is a wicked lie and it completely misunderstands what true love in any form really is.

Let me explain.

I love my two daughters more than any words could ever convey. They are my world. I simply and utterly adore them and every moment with them fills me with a joy that is indescribable. If you have children, you will know exactly what I mean.

They are breathtakingly sweet and kind, amazingly gentle and loving, brilliantly clever and funny, utterly beautiful and complete cheeky rascals, who love getting into mischief.

Their gifts and talents amaze me. Their potential is astonishing.

I am aware that they have quirks and flaws, that they make mistakes and get stuff wrong. Just like every human being that ever lived. Ever.

My love for them is complete because I love all of who they are, every aspect of them; the absolutely incredible, the more "normal," and the exhausting. I love them without condition.

If they didn't have their unique personalities, they wouldn't be **them**.

I don't think that they are "better" than any other beautiful, wonderful, precious children. That would be insane. But none of that in any way negates all the things I have just said about them.

I simply know, down to my very DNA, that I love those girls more than anything in the world; that I would do anything for them; that they are incredibly precious, unique, and deserve the very best in life.

I would guess that you found me describing my love for my children pretty straightforward to digest, entirely acceptable and your ego didn't really flare up about it. That's because we all know that it is good for parents to love their children unconditionally.

Now let me describe how I feel about me – exactly the same process as I have just done for my daughters.

As you read this next section, watch your ego. Listen to what it says; tune into how it makes you feel. The clues to your progress are found in the feelings that get thrown up in these situations; the things that cause no harm to anyone yet make you feel uncomfortable.

Look for how your ego *reacts against* what I say about me. Notice if you start to feel uncomfortable reading the words I've written. Notice how *you* feel if you say the same things to yourself about yourself.

Don't judge anything in your reactions or feelings. Just observe and consider. This is all about finding the hidden roadblocks to unlocking your natural confidence and success mindset.

I absolutely love being me. I wouldn't want to be anyone else, ever. If I could somehow go back to the time before I was born and choose to be anyone, I would, without question or hesitation, choose to be me again.

I don't simply love being me, I love the person I am. I'm awesome.

I am incredibly kind, clever, decent, funny, insightful, and charming. I love that I always have a cheeky reply or answer for anything people say to me. I really enjoy that I will often say exactly what lots of other people are thinking but are too afraid to say.

I love my analytical mind that can find amazing answers and insights.

I have talents, charm, and insight that blow me away. I literally don't know how I do some of the things that I do. I love the way I look; I'm proud of the fact that I look good and take good care of myself at the gym.

I cherish my sense of adventure and growth, the fact that I never stop growing, exploring, and continuing on my journey.

I am aware and at peace with the fact that I have flaws and quirks.

I can be too blunt; I can easily get way too focused on my work. When I really get into something, I can easily get so into it that I lose balance in my life and lose sight of other things that are really important; and that I can upset those around me with my single-mindedness.

I know I can think I'm right too much of the time and that can be seriously annoying to people around me. I can be less patient than I would like to be of those who don't want to progress and help themselves.

Despite knowing that judgement is weakness, I have to be very focused on not judging others. My ego loves me being judgmental. It is a flaw I need to work on every day.

I love myself and I love being me, both in spite of and because of, all of the good, all of the normal, and all of the "bad" that makes me who I am.

I recognize that lots of my weakness are my strengths taken to extremes; that my strengths and talents wouldn't exist without the quirks and flaws.

I love myself without condition, and that love wouldn't shift one little bit based on anyone else's opinion of me.

I don't compare myself with anyone else in any way. Why would I? Where's the benefit in that? I know I'm not perfect, but neither do I have any desire to be perfect; that would mean to remove the things that make me unique. Being perfect would mean a loss of who I am, not a gain.

I simply know, down to my very DNA, that I love myself completely; that I would do absolutely anything for me; that I am unique and wonderful and deserve the very best in life.

So how did you feel reading that section?

How did you feel saying all those great things to yourself? If saying those kind, loving, wonderful things about someone else felt right but saying them about yourself felt wrong, then you've found a piece of the bad programming that has been holding you back.

LOVING YOURSELF ISN'T VANITY, IT'S SANITY

Recognize that there's nothing normal or natural about only allowing yourself to feel, at best, neutral or, more likely, negative about yourself.

Recognize the con trick that says that being neutral or negative about yourself is what modesty and humility looks like. That's bullshit, and highly damaging bullshit at that.

Modesty and humility are not about denying all the things that make you great, wonderful, and amazing. That's just dishonest and inaccurate thinking disguised as something that the world considers good.

Humility is about seeing the truth of who you are: all the great and all the flaws. It is loving all of it but simply recognizing that your journey is to become the very best version of yourself. And seeing that that journey will never end, and nor do you want it to; each day is an adventure to explore the fullest extent of your greatness.

The reason so many self-help books, courses, and teachers fail to land their (very true) messages with you is because you have been taught this mental block that you didn't realize you had.

<u>The great teaching can't land because there's a bunch of bad programming in the way blocking it</u>. The bad programming says that to love yourself is wrong, vain, and conceited. The great teaching says that loving yourself is good and the way to confidence and success. But you want to be a good person so you block the teaching that makes you feel like you'd be doing something that you've been taught is bad.

With contradictions like that, it's little wonder that most people struggle to truly love themselves.

How can you aspire to something that you've been taught is bad and that you associate with all things negative? The only way is to start in the right place, which is to remove the bad thinking first. That's why this book is structured the way it is.

I can only teach you the right way to be confident and successful once I've shown you how to remove the bad programming that would otherwise block this teaching.

Let me be completely clear: loving yourself should be your highest aspiration. It means exactly what it says and nothing more. It is a simple feeling of love: kind, non-judgmental caring for yourself.

Just because most of the world thinks it also means vanity and arrogance doesn't make it true.

Remember the truth is the truth even if no one believes it. A lie is a lie even if everyone believes it.

And until you shed this limiting idea, you will always limit your confidence and success. In effect, most people have been taught that self-esteem is actually bad. You can now choose to put down this baggage that weighs most of the world down terribly. You no longer have to be kept trapped by that thinking.

SELF-LOVE IS THE SOURCE OF ALL OTHER LOVES

When you start to love yourself, you will see it has a profoundly positive effect on all of your relationships. If you've struggled in your relationships, this will be a big part of the reason for that.

You may have heard that you cannot truly love another until you love yourself first. And it's completely true.

But here's why it's true.

You cannot give the best of yourself to anyone or anything unless you're filled up with love from within. ***You cannot give love if you're empty of love from within to begin with.***

Your ego is likely to be flaring up right now and screaming that you are a loving person. And I'm not suggesting that's not true. But what happens is that many people unconsciously act in far less loving ways than they realize.

Let me explain.

When you love and accept yourself completely, you go into any relationship, into any interaction ***to give***, because you're already filled up with love. Your only agenda is to be you, the best you, and explore and enjoy the relationship. That means you give without any expectation of anything in return – because you don't need anything in return.

You have everything you need within you already.

You don't need the other person to "save" you, to make you feel whole, to "complete you," or anything similar. You know that you and your life are already amazing. This incredible person and the relationship **will**

add to your life, instead of being necessary to in some way save or complete your life.

But when you aren't filled up with love from within, when you struggle to love yourself, when you're running on empty in terms of the love you have inside of you, you enter into any relationship, consciously or unconsciously, **to get**: to take from the other person; to get your needs met, to have someone save you, complete you, and so on.

That's not loving without agenda, nor is it giving without agenda. The agenda is actually pretty obvious: you are in the relationship and "loving" this person *in order to get your needs met*.

How loving does that really sound? Or does it sound like a contract? How loving would you feel in response to such a contract as opposed to simply being with someone that was fully loving (by which I mean they gave love without agenda or expectation) because they were already filled up with love from within?

Can you see the difference? More importantly, can you feel the difference?

Can you see how if two people filled up with love were in a relationship, how different, how much more loving, that relationship would be?

This is true with your partner, with family, with your children, with your friends, with anyone you interact with.

Let me give you a slightly different example.

You may have seen my Instagram page (@unstoppableselfconfidence). I give the very best of myself on those posts each and every day. I receive numerous direct messages, emails, and texts from people asking me for help. And I am happy to help where I can.

I can do that without expecting anything in return because I am already filled up from within; that all stems from my unconditional love of myself.

So, through self-love, I put more love, kindness, and giving into the world, into every relationship and with every interaction.

Imagine if the whole world was filled with love from within. Imagine how different the world would look. But let's just start with one mind at a time. And today, let's make that mind yours.

HOW TO STOP SACRIFICING YOURSELF

Have you ever heard the phrase, "Don't be a martyr"?

Are you someone who feels like you always sacrifice yourself for the good of others and end up feeling stressed, underappreciated, resentful, and even angry as a result?

Have you considered that this is a role you have given yourself? That it's a role you have fallen into through bad teaching and misunderstanding healthy sacrifice?

Let me explain what I mean.

Nearly everyone is taught that sacrificing your desires, your time, your dreams, and even your happiness for others is kind, noble, and loving.

And that saying no to others, putting your needs and desires equal to or in front of others makes you selfish and bad. But this is muddled thinking that makes you a victim and quickly destroys your self-esteem.

The world is taught by default that you "should" give up the things that you want and that make you happy in order to make others happy; and that this act of giving up your happiness should in some perverse way make you proud and happy.

So, you sacrifice more and more until it becomes a habit that you stop even being aware of; until you are completely empty, with nothing left to give, miserable and worn out, which is the only end game of habitual, toxic self-sacrifice.

The wickedness of this teaching is profound. You are taught that to be a good, worthy, and decent person you must give up the things that matter to you most, as a symbol of that worthiness and decency.

There is a time and a place for sacrificing what you want for the greater good, for those you love and care about. But this should be a clear, deliberate, careful, and **conscious choice**.

It should involve balancing your own goals, needs, and desires with supporting those you love in getting theirs met. This is conscious and healthy sacrifice.

Unconscious, unhealthy sacrifice is when you become a martyr, by accident or design. It's when you don't give yourself any space or priority to meet your needs and desires, or to pursue personal fulfillment and your goals. It's when, by default and as a matter of routine, you push what you want to the side.

But the vast majority aren't aware of this choice because nearly the whole world believes that sacrifice, in and of itself, is a noble act. _And so, your identity as a good, kind person is tied in with sacrifice_. The more you sacrifice, the more decent, kind, and noble you understand yourself to be.

And if you tie your self-esteem in to the act of sacrifice, if you think that sacrificing yourself makes you a good person, what you're really saying is that your life, your needs, and your desires have no value.

This programming gives your ego another stick to beat you with every time you try to become the person you want to be and create the life you want to live.

With each attempt to focus on your dreams, your ego tells you that you're unkind, selfish, and uncaring of those around you.

You self-sabotage at every step because you feel bad, like you're doing something wrong by doing what's right for you. And so, you constantly struggle to make progress.

Until you learn to properly value yourself and your life, you will struggle to get off this hamster wheel. Until you see the difference between healthy and unhealthy sacrifice, you will sacrifice yourself on autopilot. And despite what you may think, you are not a victim; you are the perpetrator of this.

I know that saying that massively grates against everything you've been taught about what it means to be a good person, but it doesn't make it any less true. And it doesn't stop the bad teaching from destroying your self-esteem.

Your life is precious. Your dreams matter. And becoming the very best, most authentic you is the greatest gift you can give to the world. So don't feel guilty for doing what's best for you. Only then can you give your best to others.

THE ASTONISHING POWER OF LIVING AUTHENTICALLY

Everyone is born a genius, but the process of life de-geniuses them.

– R. BUCKMINSTER FULLER

You were born with greatness within you. I get that that sounds hokey, but it doesn't make it any less true.

Your greatness is unique to you. Your greatness isn't the same as anyone else's. You can only give full expression to your talents and gifts – to your greatness – by living in alignment with who you really are.

Otherwise, you literally end up being a second-rate version of someone else instead of a first-rate version of yourself.

Authenticity, then, is the key to unlocking the greatness that lies within you.

Think of authenticity as the filter that defines what comes into and stays out of your life.

When you act authentically, when you think authentically, when you live authentically, you create a filter that only allows in the right things for you: the right people, the right opportunities, the right experiences, the right possibilities, the right coincidences.

You set your incredible subconscious mind to work for you in creating your very best life.

The more of the right things you allow into your life and the more of the wrong things you keep out, the more you will live life on your terms; the more you will live a life of incredible fulfilment and joy, a life that makes complete sense to you.

You intuitively sense and see the right things to desire in your life and so the journey and the destination become the reward.

When you live inauthentically you have in effect installed the wrong filter for your life. You've installed a cheap generic filter (one that is designed for everyone instead of specifically for you) and so through unconscious thought, you filter out the incredible people, opportunities, and experiences that life puts in your path every day.

You will turn away from incredible possibilities for your life because you either won't recognize them or you will see them as wrong because they don't align with the inauthentic vision you have for your life, when your social conditioning and ego are in charge instead of the real you.

You set your incredible subconscious mind to work to create a life that doesn't fulfill you and to sabotage your success on that wrong goal. So, you don't get the real success you want and you fail at what you've been taught success "should be." And so, you think that you're a failure.

If you're exhausted, worn out, and ground down by habitually sacrificing yourself, you've effectively turned this filter off completely, and anything and everything that flows into your life is a complete jumble that makes no real sense at all.

The day you start living authentically is the day you set yourself on the right path for you. It is the day you start living life on your terms.

It is when each step, each action, each choice starts to work in concert and alignment for your greater good. It is when life starts to make sense.

The greatest freedom in life is being completely, fearlessly, and unapologetically authentic.

You drop all the baggage; throw off all the shackles, lose all the pretense. You no longer need to act, to second-guess yourself, to hide anything about yourself from anyone. It is complete and total acceptance of who you are.

You no waste time, energy, and focus on building a façade, a patchwork life made up of all the things you think you are supposed to be, do, or have. You no longer feel any need to prove yourself or your worth to a false or arbitrary standard. You embrace who you are instead of fighting against who you are.

You become still inside and at peace.

The wrong people and the wrong circumstances for you start to fall away. You make space for the right ones to flow into your life.

IMAGINE GOING THROUGH YOUR WHOLE DAY BEING UNAPOLOGETICALLY YOU

I would like you to give yourself a gift, if you want to.

I would like you to give yourself a day, just one day, where you are 100% no bullshit, no shading, no cutting corners – just completely and totally authentically you.

Imagine if just for today you took the handbrake off. You completely let go of all inhibitions, all fears, all doubts, and all thoughts of whether or not you were enough.

All concerns about the judgements people might make about you. Imagine if for today, you completely stopped giving even the smallest shit about what anyone thought of you.

If you started saying what you really thought instead of what people said you should think. If you started doing what you loved instead of what other people said was "realistic" for you.

Imagine if you started being 100% present and in the moment in your life. Not weighed down by the false baggage of your past. Not filled with fear and trepidation of what may happen in the future.

Imagine if you simply said "Fuck it. I will be me 100% without fear or apology."

What do you think that day would feel like?

Now take a moment to realize that all of this is your natural state and all I am suggesting to you is that you allow yourself to return to that natural state.

Now imagine how incredible your life would be if you lived this way every day.

That is the choice you now have. You always had it but now I have made it a conscious choice instead of an unconscious one.

What will you choose?

THINGS TO CONSIDER

- Can you see that authenticity is confidence?
- Do you feel comfortable fully expressing your talents and gifts? Or do you hide them away in case others think you are "showing off"?
- Can you see that by hiding your gifts away, you are living your life to a fraction of its real potential?
- Consider. Can you see your talents and gifts as clearly as your faults?
- Do you feel comfortable telling yourself and others that you love yourself? If not, consider why not.
- Consider that self-love is the source of all other loves; that without loving yourself first you cannot be truly loving to another.
- Do you see sacrificing yourself for the good of others as kind, decent, and noble? Have you decided to sacrifice your needs and wants consciously or indiscriminately?

CHAPTER 14

THE CAREFREE OPERATING SYSTEM

> **Being free brings a lightness, a carefree surrender to all that is happening around you, and above all, an acceptance of reality.**
>
> DEEPAK CHOPRA

When you picture the very best version of yourself, confident and successful, how do you imagine feeling as that person?

Burdened and worn down by worries, concerns, and stresses? Or relaxed, at ease, and happy? Completely carefree, giving off a great vibe, and just going with the flow of life?

People who are carefree have a wonderful energy. The way they just seem to breeze through life draws people to them. Their carefree attitude creates a natural charm and charisma.

It is a different level of confidence – a confidence not just about themselves but about life.

It is like they have discovered the magic formula to life. This is more than just the absence of worry. This is a deep state of calmness, almost serenity, no matter what is happening.

Almost everything in life and about life is better when you're relaxed and carefree. You do everything better when you're in a relaxed, carefree, calm, focused state of mind; you can access the very best of you, the best of your skills and talents.

Carefree people have problems just like everyone else.

But the difference is that carefree, confident, and successful people know that they are <u>bigger than their problems</u>. They know that they will handle whatever life puts their way. They know problems are <u>just situations to deal with</u>. And they know that their greatest benefit lies in their problems.

As a result, they are relaxed and happy with life no matter what.

But being carefree isn't some magical power that only a select few have. It is your natural state. It is within you right now and I'm going to show you exactly how to access it and <u>how to stay</u> in that state.

THE POWER OF BEING CAREFREE

*The more relaxed you are, the better you are at everything:
the better you are with your loved ones, the better you are
with your enemies, the better you are at your job, the better
you are with yourself.*

– BILL MURRAY

Take a moment and think of all the times when you have been at your absolute best. When your life has been at its best; when you just breezed through your problems and nothing could bring you down.

That's the power of being carefree. It is simultaneously how you create your best life and live your best life.

It is how you gain the fullest access to your talents and how those talents can be most easily expressed.

Being carefree is the perfect state for your authentic confidence and success in whatever you are doing.

Now, before we go on, I want to be really clear about what I mean and don't mean by "being carefree." Most people get pulled down into really unhelpful binary thinking on this that can easily derail their shift to living a carefree life.

First, being carefree is essentially being non-needy, unattached to any outcome. It means you know what you desire life to be like, but you are completely open and OK to it being different from your preconceived ideas. You don't need any particular outcome to happen even though you may desire it.

Being carefree doesn't mean that you "don't care" about people, places, your goals, key issues, etc. It means that you don't need those things to be exactly as your preconceived ideas say they "should be."

It means that your sense of well-being is based on your trust and faith in yourself and in the process of life rather than in specific circumstances being as they "should."

Think of it as the opposite of neediness. It is an openness to life, to different paths, choices, and outcomes. It is recognizing that none of us have all the answers and none us truly know 100% what is the absolute "right" way for life to be.

Second, being carefree doesn't mean being an uncaring asshole. Far from it. Being carefree means you can give the best of yourself to people, places, and issues without requiring them to be as you would choose. Instead, you give the best of yourself without condition, again because you don't need a specific outcome. You care but are not attached. You desire, but do not need.

Instead of forcing life, you work in harmony with life.

Can you feel how one way sets you free from the worry and anxiety that inevitably results from needing life to be a particular way? And how the other way inevitably causes you continual anxiety and worry?

When you stop needing life to be "just so," you can start seeing all of the options available to you instead of a small, limited set of them.

Because you are unattached to the outcome, you can ask for things that others would consider off-limits. As you are not beholden to how others will view what you do, say, or think, your choices become authentic instead of driven by a need to please or be accepted.

Because you have reached a point of being at complete peace no matter what outcome happens, you are free to say things you might not otherwise say, to ask for or even demand things you wouldn't otherwise ask for, to take risks you may have otherwise considered off-limits.

And in all of this you are able to access a level of life most never get to experience.

Let me give you a personal example to demonstrate this.

I used to be self-employed working for banks in London. It was intense work with a lot of pressure. One of people I worked with on one job was a complete pain in the ass. Big time. He was one of those people who enjoyed attempting to make others uncomfortable, miserable, and look bad. He used to set people up to fail all the time.

When I was working for this company, I had a newborn child and the economy was in a bad way. I needed the money and I felt like I needed that work. In short, I was attached to the outcome (maintaining that work). Because I was attached, because I felt that I needed the work, I accepted a lot of pretty appalling treatment that only got worse over time.

You may have been in similar situations. This continued until eventually it became unbearable.

I was in a meeting, where despite having worked my nuts off to do a piece of work exactly as this guy requested, he then immediately tore it to pieces in front of a lot of very senior people, blaming me for the "terrible" work that he had requested and signed off the previous day.

By this point I had had enough and no longer cared what the consequences were.

I met with him immediately afterwards and told him what I thought, what he had done, and that working this way was no longer acceptable at all. I said that I would be leaving the role that day unless that behavior stopped.

Because by this stage I was completely unattached to the outcome, I also said that I was being underpaid compared to my peers and treated disrespectfully – both of which were true but because of my previous neediness I hadn't spoken up about.

The result was that his demeanor changed significantly and immediately. And to be clear, I would have been OK if it hadn't and if I had needed to leave that role.

I walked out of that meeting with a changed work situation and improved financial terms. While it would be a lie to say that we had a good relationship after that, it never once returned to the previous state.

Can you see the power of becoming unattached? I'm not suggesting being reckless with the moves you make. But I am illustrating the breadth of the choices you make available to yourself when you are detached from the outcome.

The key point is that it was only when I became detached, only when I no longer emotionally needed any particular outcome that the situation changed quickly and for the better.

You may well have experienced similar situations.

EVERYTHING WORKS OUT FOR THE BEST

Everything that happens in your life, happens perfectly in order for you – and everyone involved with you – to grow exactly in the way you've needed and wanted to grow.

– NEALE DONALD WALSCH

So now you can see the power of being detached but the question is how do you learn to be detached from those things that matter to you the most?

It sounds completely counterintuitive, doesn't it?

This is why this section of the book is about (re)installing all the right ways to think, ways of thinking that help you to replace the destructive unhelpful ways that 99% of people walk around with every day.

This is something that is easy and natural once you think in the right ways instead of the wrong ways.

Attachment and need come from a sense that things should or must work out in a particular way; that if they don't work out as we perceive they must, then "bad" things will happen, that we will experience pain, and that we will lose out in some way.

But what if that isn't true? What if in fact it's impossible for you to lose out? What if the outcome that you are attached to isn't actually the best thing for you?

What if the outcome you've decided you need <u>is actually taking you away from your best life</u>?

What if the outcome that you fear and dread is <u>exactly what you need</u> to create the life you have always dreamed of?

Well, that is exactly the case.

Life always and only works out for the best. But what's best often looks different from what our limited minds can conceive.

I remember both Stephen and Andy telling me exactly this point: that by me judging situations as "bad" that I was blocking the incredible gifts that life was offering me.

That by me fighting against an outcome I was blocking up the pipes, the delivery system, that was trying to give me exactly what I needed for my highest good.

That it was not the events, people, or outcomes that were the problem. It was my judgement of them as "bad" that was.

What if, instead of needing any particular outcome, you instead simply knew what you desired the outcome to be but accepted the truth?

The truth that whatever happens works out for the best.

That you calmly and diligently worked towards creating the outcome you wanted but had no need to stress or strain because no matter what happened you knew <u>with 100% certainty</u> that whatever outcome happened was not simply OK, **but the very best thing possible** for your highest good?

Even if it looked like something bad, you could relax, knowing with calm certainty that it was the best possible thing for your life, even if the whole world saw it as something "bad."

For a long time, I fought very hard to save my marriage and my family. I had decided that breaking up our family was a disaster. I was <u>completely attached</u> to the idea that the **only** good outcome was us staying together as a family.

Eventually I came to realize that, despite the fact that it wasn't yet "officially" over, our marriage had long since ended. And I realized that I was now standing in my own way, blocking my own path to a life that worked and made sense for me; and that what I saw as a terrible outcome and had fought against was actually the very thing I needed to live my best life.

Without the divorce, I never would have gone on the journey I needed to learn how to control my mind.

I wouldn't have met Stephen and struck up the friendship I now have with him. I never would have become friends with Andy Shaw. These are the two people who have completely transformed my life and have given me so much of the knowledge I am sharing with you now. The exact knowledge I needed to live my very best life.

I never would have learned the secrets to creating the indestructible, unstoppable, natural confidence of the 1%.

I have met so many kind, decent, incredible, wonderful people directly as a result of what I once thought was the worst thing to happen to me. I have experienced friendships and kindness from expected and entirely unexpected people that I will be grateful to for the rest of my life.

Without my divorce, I never would have created *Unstoppable Self-Confidence*. You would not be reading this book now. All the people who have contacted me to tell me how incredibly their lives have been changed as a result of what I teach, would not have had that experience.

And that is just a *tiny fraction* of the incredible benefit to my life directly as a result of the "worst" thing to ever happen to me. I could write pages more of all the wonderful and amazing experiences I have had directly as result of what happened, but you can see the point.

Everything works out for the best, even if it looks like the very worst thing to happen to you.

The only way it doesn't work out for the best is if you decide to not look for the benefit and value to you in the experience that you're having; to not calm your mind and see the possible ways it could (not definitely will, just could) work out for the best.

Being attached to particular outcomes was a very deep-rooted way of thinking for me. I have put in huge work and still do today to be conscious of any time I feel the need (not desire) to have things turn out the way I have decided they "should."

By letting go (not giving up), I can get on with creating my best life, without fear, anxiety, or stress. I can be open to something way bigger and better and more abundant than the dreams I have conceived as possible. And so, my journey becomes faster, easier, and more fun.

How much of your precious life have you wasted seeking to control situations, events, and people around you?

Trying to force, push, or make them be "just so," as you have decided they "should" be.

There is one thing and only one thing you have the ability to control 100%, and that is your own mind.

For everything else, control is an illusion.

And yet so many people spend almost no time learning to master control of themselves and instead waste huge time and effort trying to control external situations and people.

They fear that if the world isn't just so, if other people aren't as they should be, that somehow their life will be diminished, compromised, and unhappy.

And they do this without seeing the irony that seeking to control the uncontrollable is the very thing that pretty much guarantees you feeling anxious and unhappy.

<u>The answer is to focus on the truth – the truth that no matter what happens, that life always works out for the best for you.</u>

That life is always and only giving you exactly what you need to become who you want to be and to create the life you want to live.

This shift in perspective sets you free of being attached to set outcomes or fearing anything bad happening. You no longer fear external events or what others may say or do. You are no longer attached to anything being the way it "should" be.

Because you understand the truth that it is never something to fear, it is something to help you. Then you can start to calmly respond instead of reacting in fear or anxiety; to work with life instead of against it.

And you can let go of the need to control anything other than your own mind. You realize that is working against you becoming the very best you and creating your best life.

Confident and successful people have no attachment to specific outcomes, have no need for things to be "just so."

All they have to do is look for the benefit, for the ways in which that situation could (remember not definitely will, just could) work out for the best for them.

By feeding their subconscious mind with all the possible ways it could work out for the best instead of all the possible ways it could be terrible, they set their incredible subconscious mind to work to make it work out for the best.

JUST A SITUATION TO DEAL WITH

So much of living carefree is simply about replacing inaccurate, harmful, and destructive thoughts with accurate, natural helpful ones.

When problems arise, when challenges come into your life, having your default thinking working the right way, instead of the wrong way, means that you deal with those problems and challenges with ease.

To the outside world, it will look like you don't experience problems at all, like life seems effortless for you. And to an extent that is true.

But the real truth is simply that you know the truth. You understand that life is on your side and that each problem or *challenge is simply a situation to deal with*.

So, here's exactly how you deal with a problem or challenge the next time one comes up. This is problem solving the natural way.

Step 1 is to slow down and calm your mind, to take a moment to check you are in control of your thoughts and not your ego.

Step 2 is to remind yourself of the truth that no matter how bad things look, you know your life always works out for the best and this situation is being presented to you for your highest good.

Step 3 is to consider all the possible ways that this situation could work out for the best for you: all the lessons you could learn; all the skills, strength, and wisdom you could acquire; all the possible changes that could make your life better. They are always there, even if you can't see them at first.

<u>Step 4</u> is to decide what your desired outcome is – to recognize that this may or may not be the best possible outcome. But you know in your own mind what you would like to happen. Check that you are in a state of allowing other outcomes to happen and not attached to one specific outcome needing to happen.

<u>Step 5</u> is to consider all your options to achieve your desired outcome, no matter how realistic or unrealistic they seem. And then after reasonable consideration, move forward in a diligent, workmanlike way to bring about the desired outcome.

As you work on the outcome you would like, you remain open and receptive to the lessons you are being given; you allow your mind to consider the question "I wonder how this will work out for the best for me?" as you work on your desired outcome. You remain open to a different outcome.

You don't judge what is happening by appearances, but instead stay grounded in the underlying truth that this is for your highest good.

You deal with whatever happens in a diligent way, doing all you can to bring about the best outcome. You look for every lesson, every opportunity, knowing that it is there. You learn the lessons and apply them.

Then, no matter what, you move forward stronger, wiser, and better equipped, with new skills and experiences and new opportunities that have only been acquired through the problem or challenge you have faced.

This is natural problem solving and it is what makes you unstoppable.

THE SECRET TO LIVING CAREFREE

I want to introduce you to one of the biggest secrets to confidence, success, and a great life in general.

I have deliberately put this in the later stages of the book because it goes so much against the grain of what everyone thinks is "the way" that nearly everyone dismisses it straightaway.

And I did too.

When Andy taught me this at first, I'll be honest that I dismissed it out of hand. I judged it instead of considering it. And as a result, I blocked myself from having one of the most powerful mindset tools there is.

I did this despite Andy being my friend and mentor, someone I trust completely.

But it is without doubt one of the most important concepts there is to a successful and confident life.

As I tell you this, watch your ego try to dismiss it as being too simple, too "woo-woo," too...anything.

That's what our egos do: if it's too simple, it's dismissed and the value is lost. If it's too complicated, our egos say you have to be "special" to get it and so it gets blocked. And the value is lost.

So, decide not to judge; instead, simply consider. Because it is in that consideration that the power of what I'm describing will be fully revealed to you. And it is in your judgement that this power will get taken away and lost to you by your ego dismissing this concept without consideration.

Your greatest power comes from surrender.

Let me repeat that. Your <u>greatest</u> power comes from surrender.

Not just more power, not just more confidence, not simply more success, but your very greatest confidence, power, and success comes from complete surrender.

The problem is that nearly the whole world "knows," and so no longer questions, that surrender is ultimate weakness. Earlier in this book I talked about how judgement was weakness and observation was power. Well, this is a perfect example of why that is.

Once you make a judgement about something, all learning stops. You have reached a decision point and a decision point means you shift from your mind being open to closed.

You stop thinking; you stop considering. That judgement becomes locked away as a fact, untouchable and unchallengeable. Your mind's reticular activating system then filters in (makes visible to you) facts and data that support that decision, and filters out (makes *invisible* to you) facts and data that don't support that decision.

And you have made or been taught hundreds of things that you "know" that you are often not even aware of. I dedicated the first section of this book to removing the biggest and worst of these.

But this is why so many people stick with ways of living, ways of thinking, and ways of behaving that cause them so much harm.

They stopped considering things that they "know," despite that it no longer (and maybe never did) served them in any way.

Do you know that Mark Twain quote? *"It ain't what you don't know that gets you into trouble. It's what you know for sure that just ain't so."*

The whole world "knows" surrender is bad, terrible, complete weakness and so misses out on the most powerful weapon, the most powerful tool they have.

When I finally learned the power of surrender it blew me away. I was literally shocked and stunned by the power it unleashed within me to deal with anything and everything that came my way.

All of our pain, all of our sadness, upset, regret, anxiety, and fear ALL stem from resistance to what is and what may happen in the future.

And the problem with that is that it drains your creative energy, your power to not simply deal with any challenges in your life but to create a life on your terms.

When you, instead, accept what is and surrender to what will be, you free up your creative energy to be directed to solving any challenges and into creating your best life. The more you accept and surrender, the greater your power to create will be.

No longer are you burdened by your past: you surrender and accept that what happened, happened; that it happened for the best possible reason.

No longer do you fear the future. You surrender to the truth that whatever will be, will be. You accept fully and completely that you will do 100% of what you are able and prepared to do to bring about the outcome you wish to see. If that is not enough, then it is not enough and you will know that life has bigger and better plans for you, no matter what appearances suggest.

You relax into the uncertainty of life, knowing it is nothing to fear. Instead, it is the journey of your life, and something to be enjoyed in the adventure.

When you do all this, you reach your ultimate power, where you transform pain and difficulty, stress and anxiety, into serenity and peace. And in doing so, you access 100% of your creative power instead of the tiny fraction that remains for most. Because most people direct their creative energy towards inflaming their worries and anxiety.

You no longer need to fight or resist others, at least not in the way most of the world understands it. You are instead playing an entirely different game.

This doesn't mean you are passive, a pushover, with everyone able to trample all over you and take advantage of you. Quite the opposite. Instead, by freeing you and your incredible mind from the pain and suffering caused by attachment and all the "shoulds," you unleash all of its incredible power towards creating the outcome you want.

When I first learned this, I went through everything that I felt any pain, anger, stress, anxiety, or resentment about. Things in the past, things in the present, things in the future; things that had had a massive impact on me and things that had seemed small but I had carried with me for a long time. I fully and completely surrendered to each and every one of them.

I surrendered to:

- past mistakes.
- the pain I had caused others.
- the pain others had caused myself.
- the resentment I held towards people who had treated me badly.
- the possibility that I could lose access to my children.
- the destruction of the life that I had built up.
- the loss of my family as a unit.
- the loss of the financial position I had worked very hard to create.
- the outcome of the divorce, whatever it may be.
- the pain that my children were going through.
- the fact that I may or may not ever get married again or meet someone I loved again.

I accepted and surrendered to the fact that these things had happened, were happening now, or could happen in the future. Surprisingly, I often found the smaller things more difficult to let go of than some of the bigger things.

Now, here's what interesting. The moment I find what I'm resisting and surrender to it, I instantly feel completely at peace and serene. And I get an incredible rush of energy, like my mind has been suddenly fully opened and a flood of creative inspiration and ideas come flowing in.

My focus switches in a moment from "what could go wrong" to complete peace. I relax into the uncertainty and allow my subconscious mind to do its work.

Because I know (properly know) that everything (that is, absolutely everything) works out for the best for me, <u>then what is there to resist, to fight against</u>? Take a few moments to think about that. If you come to know this, think of all the pain and discomfort that no longer has any place in your life.

Then all that's left is peace, acceptance, serenity, and adventure. You're excited about what may happen, because it's all for the very best.

Every time I do this, my subconscious mind comes up with incredible ideas, solutions, answers, strategies, and tactics that seem so incredibly simple and obvious when they arrive but had been completely hidden to me before I surrendered. It is like a curtain being pulled back and all the greatest knowledge suddenly being revealed to me just as I need it.

Now I remain always aware of what is going on inside me. Each and every time I feel any pain or resistance, it is a signal to look inside and see what I am resisting or fighting against. Any pain or bad feelings mean that there is something I need to accept and surrender to. I look for it, consider it, and then surrender completely to it.

GRATITUDE CHANGES EVERYTHING

If the only prayer you said in your whole life was "thank-you" that would be enough.

– MEISTER ECKHART

It's amazing how one simple action can change so much in a person's life.

The simple daily practice of examining your life and taking a little time each day to be grateful for all that you have, all the wonderful things in your life, for the simple experience of being here, alive, in the world.

The transformative power of gratitude is astonishing.

You've probably read or seen quotes about gratitude. You may well have thought that it sounds like a good idea before your ego distracted you away to focus on something else.

But have you made this part of your life?

Or did you dismiss it as some hippie bullshit that only weirdos do? Well, here's why gratitude matters.

Your mind is a perceptual machine. You take in almost incalculable amounts of data all day, every day; so much data, in fact, that only a tiny fraction of what you take in ever makes it to your conscious awareness.

What that means is that our minds are filters, filtering in and out of our conscious awareness the things that are most relevant to us.

How is what's most relevant defined? <u>By your dominant thoughts</u>.

So, if you're focused on all the things that make you negative, angry, or resentful, your mind will take the mass of data and filter out the things (experiences, people, events, opportunities, etc.) that don't align with that focus.

So, you get presented with more and more stuff that makes you feel angry, negative, and resentful.

However, if you fill you mind daily with all the wonder, joy, love, incredible people, wonderful memories, and amazing opportunities that are there, your mind will show you more of that.

Both are facts; both are part of your experience. But you can choose which ones you get to experience more of. Can you see how this works?

Here's what's interesting. When you focus on gratitude, you start to see more of the incredible possibilities and opportunities right in front of you. Because you've programmed your mind through gratitude to see them instead of dismissing them.

And so, you get more and more to be grateful for.

We communicate with and we instruct our subconscious minds through our dominant thoughts and feelings.

Most people do this by accident. I've now shown you how to do this on purpose. That's why focusing on what you're grateful for isn't just some new age hippie thing. It's how you get what you want on purpose.

Now, can you see how carefree this one way of thinking can make you? To know that you have in your own mind the power to create wonderful, incredible experiences, people, and opportunities into your life simply by spending some time reflecting on and enjoying all the great things that have already happened to you?

This isn't hard work (don't let your ego fool you here). This is some of the most enjoyable time you can have, to create yet more of the most enjoyable things you can ever have.

When I first created my gratitude list, I could literally feel my focus shifting, slowly at first, like big slabs of rock grinding against the ground. But as I built momentum on this and experienced firsthand its incredible power, it became easier and easier.

Now it is a way of life. Now not a day goes by when I don't take some time to consider all the things (big and small) that I feel grateful for.

It's so easy to focus by default on your problems, but this process resets your focus fast. It's helped me feel carefree, serene, happy, and relaxed day to day. I walk around feeling blessed because I direct my focus on all the things that I feel incredibly blessed with.

It actually becomes hard to stay in a bad mood or a negative state for very long. And my life has become wonderful as a result.

There's no rocket science about how you do this (watch how your ego likes to look for a silver bullet answer and dismisses anything that feels straightforward and normal). <u>The breakthrough comes from actually doing it.</u>

I can show you this and explain the truth of how powerful this is, how this will benefit you in incredible ways. But only you can decide to apply it.

The best way to shift to a grateful mindset is to create a gratitude list – a list of all the things big and small and in between that you are grateful for.

I'm going to guess that you've heard about doing this before and that most likely you've dismissed it or tried it very briefly and decided that it didn't work. Well, the difference is that you now understand why it works and why it is so important to living a carefree, confident, successful life on your terms.

So do this on your phone, laptop, or with paper and pen – whatever feels right to you. How you do it doesn't matter. **Actually doing it does.**

I use a note-taking app on my phone for this because it syncs with all my other devices. That way I can update it and read through it from my computer at home, on my iPad, or on my phone during the day.

Take a moment to think about all the things you have to be grateful for. These don't have to be massive things. The small moments carry as much weight as the massive moments do. I have moments of my daughters dancing with great big smiles on their faces, hearing them giggle or call me Daddy for the first time, being excited to see me when I pick them up from school. How grateful I am for finding two incredible teachers in Andy and Stephen, for my family and friends, for growing up in Australia, for great nights out with good friends, for the places I've been able to travel to, for all the kindness expected and unexpected people showed me during and after my divorce.

I'm grateful for my home. I'm grateful for the journey I'm on with *Unstoppable Self-Confidence*, for finding my purpose, for great relationships I've had in the past, for the sense of excitement I feel for my life to come.

Just let this flow out of you. It may take a few moments to get going – that's OK. But just start.

By starting, you unblock the pipes and you start to remember all the incredible things that bless your life but your ego has hidden away from you and parked behind your problems.

When I first did this, it took me a little bit of time to get started. But once I did, I actually found it hard to stop. I think I ended up with around 100 things when I first got going; the number doesn't matter, the feeling of calm, gratitude, and the realization of all the wonderful things in your life does, so keep at this.

Each day as part of my morning routine, I spend some time looking back over my list, reviewing and remembering (and being grateful for) my journal of all the incredible moments I would have otherwise lost. I actively scan my life for new things to put on the list. I scan for my blessings not my problems. And so, my lens, my perspective on life, is transformed.

I can get very emotional when I read my list.

When you first do this, your ego will try to tell you that you don't have much (or anything) to be grateful for; that this is silly, a waste of time; that you have more important things to do. These are lies to distract you from taking the very steps that will speed you on your way to the life you want. See this for what it is: a trap your ego is setting for you to block your progress.

One word of warning here. If you don't decide, after reading this, to go and create this list today, you're unlikely to do it. So now (yes right now) put this book down and go and create your gratitude list.

There is nothing more important for you to do today.

How did you get on? Did you create your list?

If you did, how did you feel afterwards? Did you realize all the incredible things that you already had in your life? Do you feel somehow lighter, more at peace with the world, realizing all of the incredible things you have in your life?

If you didn't do it and just read on, slow down and consider why you did that. Why did you decide not to give yourself the opportunity to experience these wonderful feelings, this wonderful sense of peace and serenity, this pathway to being carefree?

Beware your ego rushing you past the point of taking action and assuming (falsely) that because you've read this you know it; that because you've read this before and tried it once you know it and "it didn't work." These statements, and many more just like it, are the traps that your ego sets to stop you making progress. So, consider, if you want to, going back and giving this a go.

As you make acceptance, surrender, and gratitude a way of life, something magical starts to happen: you no longer feel bad. It's not that you're trying or forcing not feeling bad, you simply don't.

As things happen, as any issues or problems arise, your new default is acceptance of what is and surrendering to what will come. You know life works out for the best so you know that even if something looks bad, it will be of benefit to you. So, you can relax into the uncertainty, then search for, find, and apply the benefits. There is no room in your thinking for feeling bad because it's a waste of your time.

By keeping your mind focused on all you have to be grateful for, you program your incredible subconscious mind to find more and more things for you to be grateful for. And so, your life fills up with wonderful, incredible experiences, people, and things. And as a result, negative feelings are just caught and dissolve.

Each time a negative thought comes in, you remember that every thought helps you or harms you and so you calmly observe your thoughts, assessing and weighing each one for whether it is helping you or not.

When you start to the see the truth that harmful thoughts are working against you, they become very easy to drop.

This isn't denying your feelings – far from it. It is getting as close to them as possible. It is looking at, feeling, and understanding <u>every feeling</u> you have. But it is about directing and focusing your emotions – the powerful tools you have in your armory – to work and fight for you, not against you.

So, feel all your feelings. But become aware of when you <u>indulge</u> instead of simply <u>process</u> your negative feelings.

WHY FEEL BAD

Take a moment and consider the question I asked you in an earlier chapter: Why feel bad?

What is the value in feeling bad about anything?

How does feeling bad, guilty, or ashamed IN ANY WAY help you, those you think you have hurt, or the wider world?

The challenge is that society thinks and so has programmed nearly everyone to feel bad about an incredible range of things: for getting something wrong, for saying the wrong things, for upsetting others, for sexual desires, for prioritizing yourself, for being "selfish," for desiring money, and a million other things like it.

These are all forms of "should" and, as a result, most people spend most of their time feeling in some way bad. It is a tragedy. But that tragedy arises because we are not taught to be conscious of our feelings, to be the observer of our feelings and so have the choice over what we feel.

As they've been growing up, I've been observing and then catching all the different ways my daughters are being exposed to the subtle but extremely toxic sense that they "should" feel bad about all kinds of things.

How they are taught to keep adding to the catalogue of things that they "should" feel bad about and bad about themselves for.

Recently one of my daughters had an argument with one of her friends. They both said some things that were hurtful to each other. I was conscious enough to realize that this was an important lesson for her – so I asked her why she was feeling bad.

She told me she felt like she was a bad person because of what she said and that she felt bad because maybe her friend no longer liked her.

I got her to slow her mind down and consider how feeling bad made the situation better in any way.

How did feeling bad help her, help her friend, or help anyone else?

I asked her to think about whether it made it easier for her to move forward and do the things that would help everyone, or more difficult because her energy was being used up with feeling bad.

I asked her to consider that she could choose to contact her friend and apologize for her part in their argument and for the things she said; that in all likelihood, if she did, they would be friends and on good terms again soon.

I reminded her that she could be conscious of what she did and aware that she didn't like the result and so choose to not do it again.

I told her that she wasn't required to feel bad for some set amount of time to show that she cared; that this was a lie that would trap and hurt her.

I saw the weight of feeling bad lift off her; I saw her smile again as she saw the truth. And shortly afterwards, she and her friend made up.

The reason for telling you this story is to show how easy it is to default to feeling bad, even when you know it holds no value or benefit for you.

Whenever I need to discipline my daughters in any way or when anything goes "wrong," I make sure that they understand that they do not need to feel bad, that feeling bad has no place in what's happening.

When they talk to me about things that happen at school, or with their friends or in any situation at all, we talk through how the purpose of the experience is to learn a lesson. It is not, never was, and never will be to feel bad. And within a few moments, I see them become conscious again of a previously unconscious choice.

I can almost physically see them put down the baggage that they were in danger of picking up. I quickly see the sparkle return to their eyes and the smiles to their faces.

They are given time, space, and support to process their feelings but not to indulge negative feelings. They are learning to ask themselves if they are choosing to feel bad or if they have gone unconscious. And it is one of my greatest joys to watch them snap themselves out if it quickly and naturally.

Each time they do this, they are learning to question what society says they "should" feel. And so, they are developing incredible mental and emotional strength naturally and without effort.

I have seen their mental and emotional strength grow hugely as a result. They understand increasingly (this lesson will continue) that **all these experiences are there for them to grow from and not to feel bad from**.

Remember, your default state is the state you're most often in.

So, this is helping them naturally create a default state of happiness and not feeling bad. And you can do the same.

All from simply being conscious and becoming aware of your thoughts.

THE NATURAL WAY TO THINK POSITIVELY

I want to cover one of the most important ways of being carefree, and that is *natural positive thinking*. Andy taught me this and it is without doubt the master key to thinking positively by default and in a way that actually creates the success that you desire.

Pretty much everyone will tell you that in order to be happy, in order to achieve, that you need to think positively.

The problem is that they don't tell you *how to think positively*.

The way most of the world is taught to thinking positively is likely to result in complete failure for 99% of people.

That's because it goes against our natural way of thinking and so requires great effort to sustain it. And that effort ultimately wears you down and wears you out.

So, despite that nearly the whole world says positive thinking is a good thing, the current way of teaching is actually sabotaging your confidence and success. "Positive thinking" in the way nearly everyone teaches it, actually adds to your doubts rather than creating the platform for success.

As counterintuitive as it may sound, the key to thinking positively naturally is not to try to think positively. Instead, <u>the key is the removal of negative thoughts</u>. Then all that is left are positive thoughts.

This is what the 1% do naturally (or rather, never had programmed out of them), even if they call it positive thinking. Remember that there is a very big difference between knowing something and being able to teach it.

And you already do this too in the areas of your life where you are already successful and where you already achieve your goals. Maybe it's in your career, maybe it's in your relationship, maybe it's as a parent.

Slow down and consider: In those areas of your life where you are already successful, how much time and effort do you put into thinking positively? How much time do you really spend straining to think positively in those aspects of your life?

Or are those areas simply characterized by an absence of negative thoughts?

Let me give you a really simple example to illustrate the point. Don't let your ego dismiss this because it's such a simple example. The process of confidence and success is the same, no matter whether the goal is massive or mundane.

This is your ego trying to distract you away for the fact that you are already successful and confident in key areas of your life. All you need to do is apply that mindset to the areas where you would like to see change.

Let's say you've decided to go the supermarket to get some food. How much time do you spend thinking positively about that goal? How much effort do you put into thinking positively, pumping yourself up, telling yourself that "You can do this," that "failure is not an option"?

Or do you simply just go to the shops, calmly, diligently, in a workmanlike way, and just get on with it?

Your mindset in that goal isn't characterized by lots of positive thoughts. It is characterized by **an absence of doubt**. And so, you succeed without effort.

You do not need positive thinking; you simply need to silence the voice in your head (your ego) that seeks to fill your mind with doubts and negative thoughts.

Right now, I'm guessing your ego is saying something like, "Well going to the shops is easy, what about for the big stuff?" Well, it's exactly the same mindset, your natural success mindset, that you need for the big stuff as for the small stuff.

Here's how you do this for the big stuff, how you create the same success mindset that you have for going to the shops, to finding your perfect partner, to creating financial success, to achieving any big goal at all.

You give up trying to think positively. You instead recognize that natural positive thinking and so confidence and success comes from *the removal of doubt*.

I put no effort at all into thinking positively. I literally never, ever tell myself that "I've got this," that "I can do this," or anything remotely similar.

Where I do put huge effort is into finding and dissolving any unhelpful doubts. I observe my thoughts and examine each one for value. I look for any areas where I feel doubt. I look for whether those doubts help me in any way; if they are showing me anything helpful or are just obstacles and roadblocks my ego is putting in my way.

Sometimes the doubts do have value: sometimes they are revealing important questions I haven't yet considered; data that I don't yet have that is necessary to move forward in whatever way is best; questions that if answered would get me to a better outcome more quickly.

Other times they are valueless, non-specific doubts like "You've never done this before," "You're not an expert," and so on. I just observe the doubts that come up, in a detached, calm way. I don't fight or resist them;

I let them come, and I shine a light on them. I have no fear of them. In many ways, I look forward to finding them because each one I find and remove speeds me on my way.

When I see that a doubt has no value or benefit to me at all, it simply dissolves. It has nothing to offer me at all, except a limit, a constraint on my ability to create the life I desire. It has no truth and so becomes the easiest thing in the world to ignore.

When I first decided to write this book, my ego instantly threw a tidal wave of doubts at me. It went into complete overdrive at first. At the time, I was heavily in debt, had just gone through a divorce, I had (and still have) no formal training relevant to what this book is about. I have never written a book before, never had a book published before, never sold a book before. I was completely unknown in this space. I had no platform in terms of contacts, brand, or experience related to creating a business in this space.

I knew the doubts would flow in from my ego. I calmed my mind and accepted that my ego would do this. I didn't fight or resist it happening. I examined each doubt and looked at it calmly and accurately without needing to be right or wrong. My only focus was on finding what would help me.

Yes, I had no experience, but no one is born experienced. No one who is succeeding in anything started with all the experience they needed. Social media (Instagram in particular) was an easy way for me to start to find my audience and share some of the knowledge I wanted to share. I could see what level of engagement I would get, and learn to hone my writing style. It was a simple and easy way to start to gain the experience and exposure I needed.

Yes, I had no formal qualifications or training, but the very best teachers I had found in many areas of my life were the best precisely because they weren't constrained by mainstream thinking. So, this wasn't a doubt that held true.

Yes, I hadn't written a book before, but that was a process. I could research great ways of how to write a book and get on with it.

Yes, I had no contacts, but I knew I could research and reach out to relevant people. I knew that by building my Instagram following, gaining contacts would become easier and easier; that having a big social presence would give me the platform I needed and open doors for me.

Yes, I was heavily in debt. But that meant my social life would be pretty constrained for some time, which gave me the perfect opportunity to throw myself into writing the book and learning all I needed to learn to get started.

Yes, I don't have the writing skills of some other authors but I knew one of my greatest skills was making things accessible in a way that actually created change in people. I had done this many times in my previous career.

I went through this process with each doubt that arose. Each doubt got explored for value and then dissolved and/or answered. Soon enough, and without pain or struggle, I was left without any real doubts. And that meant I was simply able to just get on with it.

Writing the book just became a process, something to do, rather than something I needed to think positively about.

Can you see the difference between this and what most of the world calls positive thinking? More importantly, can you feel the difference?

The journey was the removal of doubt so that all that is left is positive thought by default. No resistance, no fighting against, no stress or strain. Just observation and consideration for value.

THINGS TO CONSIDER

- Can you see that by being carefree, by living in a calm, relaxed state, you allow the fullest expression of your talents and gifts?

- Consider that being carefree doesn't mean that you don't care. It means that you are unattached to any specific outcome.

- Consider that being carefree means that your sense of well-being comes from you trusting yourself and that you trust life to always work out for the best.

- Can you see how when you stop needing life to work out 'just so," that you open yourself up to new options, to new possibilities?

- Consider that everything always works out for the best – that it is only your judgement of something as bad that blocks this.

- Consider how when you know this and live it as a way of life, how much more easily you can relax into the uncertainty of life.

- Consider that the only thing you have 100% control over is your own mind.

- Can you see that your greatest power comes from surrender?

- Consider: Is there any value in you feeling bad about anything?

CHAPTER 15

THE SECRET METHOD FOR GETTING WHAT YOU REALLY WANT

> Life punishes the vague wish and rewards the specific ask.
>
> TIM FERRISS

Do you know what you want?

This seems like such a simple and straightforward question and it is. But because it's such a simple and straightforward question, **very** few people actually take the time to consider it properly.

When I ask people if they know what they want, nearly all instinctively and <u>without thought</u> say, "Yes."

But when I ask them what it is, they either tell me a whole list of things that they don't want <u>or</u> what they think they should want <u>or</u> they will list vague things like "to be rich," "to be happy," "financial freedom," "more time," "to be less busy."

So, they think they know what they want but the truth is that they only at best have a vague idea, a sense of what they don't want, or are trapped by social conditioning and haven't tuned into their authentic desires.

As a result, they cannot create success (because they don't specifically know what success is) or they self-sabotage because their subconscious knows that the "success" they are trying to create isn't what they really want.

Can you see, <u>can you feel</u>, how not truly knowing what you want works against you, undermines your efforts and sabotages your success?

Until you know what you do want, in detail, how can you go about creating it? How do you start creating something <u>that you don't want</u>? How can you get inspired to create a life you're not actually passionate about, only one that you've been told you **should** want?

CREATING A LIFE ON MY TERMS

A couple of years ago at the end of my divorce, I realized that I had no idea what I truly wanted. My divorce was complete and I now had the opportunity to create a new life, a life that made complete sense to me – a life that I would truly love living.

A life on my terms.

The only problem was that I didn't actually know what I wanted my life to look like <u>at all</u>. All I knew was that I wanted life to be very different from how it had been in the past. But I had fallen into the trap that so many people get caught by.

Non-specific, vague fantasies; not wanting more of the same.

But that does you absolutely no good whatsoever. *And it was doing me absolutely no good whatsoever*.

I had essentially a blank sheet of paper in front of me to create whatever I wanted but I realized that I needed to be clear and precise about what I wanted if I was to have any chance of creating it.

I didn't know what I wanted any new partner to be like: what qualities they would have; what their personality would be like; what their interests would be; what they would look like; what their current situation would be, etc.

I didn't know what I wanted my lifestyle to be like: I didn't know what I wanted my working life to look like; what kind of work I wanted to do; how much I wanted to work; if I wanted to continue with a traditional career or do something completely different; how much free time I wanted; how much I ideally wanted to be around for my daughters (a lot, but I needed to be more specific); how many holidays I wanted to have; what kind of holidays; what kind of car I wanted.

Beyond wanting to be "financially free," I didn't know what I wanted my financial situation to be. I didn't even know what financial freedom looked like to me beyond a vague idea of replacing my current income. What was "enough" money to me? What was "rich" to me?

Side note: This chapter and the next one on finding your life purpose are based on and inspired by the brilliant Life Design Getaway course by Andy Shaw as well as the detailed process I went through with Stephen. If you want to understand this process in a lot more detail, I highly recommend you buy Andy's Life Design Workshop.

I sat down and watched a video program from Andy called the Life Design Workshop, which goes through how to design your life so that you actually go and create it. I spent a good part of my time with my coach Stephen working through my designs in a lot of detail.

Because I wanted to make sure they really were _my_ designs.

Up until that point, I had spent so much of my life working incredibly hard to create the life that I thought I should live and it had left me empty, exhausted, divorced, and heavily in debt. Now it was my time to create a life that made sense to me.

I went through every aspect of my life and thought about what I wanted it to look like. I considered it all in great detail.

I let it all pour out of me, everything I wanted, everything I dreamed of, without any constraint. Nothing was off-limits; nothing was out of bounds. This wasn't about being what the world called "realistic."

Fuck that.

It didn't matter if the whole world thought I was wrong, mad, or bad for what I desired. This was me giving myself complete and total freedom, for the first time since I was a child, to just say what I wanted in life.

I wrote it all down, considered it, tweaked it. I played around with what I had written and tweaked any bits that on reflection didn't feel quite right. I added in any bits that were missing.

I went through them in my sessions with Stephen and he gave me some incredible tools and insights into how to create these designs. I got him to challenge me to make sure that I wasn't falling into the trap of being "realistic," knowing that my ego would look to get me to play small.

I got him to challenge me to make sure my designs were what I wanted, all of what I wanted, and nothing but what I wanted.

In the end I had a list of around 80 things that I wanted, covering all aspects of my life.

Since creating my list and going through the Life Design process, I have achieved about 30% of the things I wrote down. And at a guess about another 30%–40% are well on their way.

And the remaining 30%–40% have either started to happen or have fallen away because I'm not sure I really want them anymore.

Some of these things are massive, huge, incredible. Others would probably appear to be far more mundane and low-key to anyone else but have, individually and collectively, made a big difference to my day-to-day quality of life.

Many of the designs have turned out way, way, way bigger than I expected or dared to dream at the time, which always reminds me how, even after going through all of this, our egos still tempt us to play small.

I'm really not kidding when I say that our potential is essentially unlimited.

But I have made exponentially more progress towards the life of my dreams and gotten far more of what I wanted in the last couple of years than in the rest of my life combined.

All from simply knowing what I wanted and reconnecting with the natural process for creating my life by design – the same process we all instinctively knew as children but was buried (not lost) under layers of bad teaching and backwards thinking.

The same process that Andy and Stephen showed me and that I will show you shortly.

GOAL SETTING AND FANTASIES VS. LIFE DESIGNS

Before I show you the step-by-step process for getting exactly what you want in life, I want to explain why, almost certainly, everything you've read and learned about goal setting, the law of attraction, and success hasn't really worked for you.

Why, despite following exactly what you read, it hasn't really made much of a difference.

Success teaching broadly falls into two big categories that I label "goal setting" and "fantasizing."

Goal setting takes something amazing (looking to get what you desire) and then finds a superb method for killing those dreams dead, usually at the first step. Ninety-nine percent of people who teach goal setting manage to turn your dream life into hard work and remove all the fun, all the joy, and all the pleasure. And at the same time, they manage to find all kinds of ways, both time-tested and newly invented, to put evermore limits on what you go after, to be evermore "realistic" so that what you end up going after isn't something that inspires you in any way. **AT ALL**.

So, there's no fun, it's all hard work, and you end up being so "realistic" (which means playing small) that all of that hard work isn't even for a result or outcome that you want.

And then they wonder why 99% of people completely fail at their "process for success."

Let's say for example that you want to write a book that will change the world. The "standard" goal setting approach immediately tells you to get "specific" and "realistic." Both those steps in this process really mean play small, shrink your horizons, don't aim for something big because you'll fail and be disappointed.

So, you write out a plan (hard work and inspiration reduced) for creating your book, for doing all the research, for doing the book outline, etc. Then you plan out how much time it "should" take you to write each chapter (second massive trap right there), and that when you miss each deadline you feel bad, you feel like success is a little further away, you feel a little bit more like this isn't realistic for you.

To counter that feeling, the standard process then tells you to break it down into smaller chunks and measure those (more hard work), to hustle, to decide how much you really want this, to work hard, to even fake it until you make it...

They ignore the fact that if you've never written a book before you have <u>absolutely no idea AT ALL of how long it takes to write a book</u>. And so, measuring this and beating yourself up because you missed a self-imposed deadline that has no experience behind it is completely fucking mental.

Soon enough, that dream, that goal you were excited about, is soon feeling like a complete nightmare, utterly hard work, no fun, and forever reducing results.

Soon enough, you feel like giving up and then you decide that you've failed at this and it isn't for you. After all, you missed all these deadlines, you didn't enjoy the process, you didn't make the progress you measured yourself against.

The only reason to do any of this is **because you doubt your success**, to impose deadlines on yourself because without them you "know" you won't make progress – which again feels like hard work.

Then, after the massive and widespread failure of these goal setting techniques, a number of new teachers come along with the "law of attraction" teaching.

Now I want to be clear that there is underlying truth in the law of attraction – it is simply that many of the teachers, without intending to, have included some massive bugs in the way it is taught which completely undermines your ability to make it work for you.

For those of you who are not new age or spiritual in any way, don't get distracted or put off by this. I will explain shortly how and why, no matter whether you believe in all things new age or indeed **none of them at all**, how this process works for you no matter what.

The law of attraction states that you decide what you desire and get into "vibrational alignment" with that desire by believing it is possible and by being grateful for it coming into your life.

 Lots of this is great, but if that was enough there would be huge numbers of people manifesting their desires right now. But there aren't and you may well be one of them.

Remember that there is a very, very big difference between people knowing what to do and <u>being able to teach what to do</u>.

And so, for many people, the law of attraction remains in the realm of fantasies; it's a process that many would love to be true, <u>but doubt to be really true</u>.

They increasingly focus their effort on "getting into vibrational alignment" and on "wanting it enough" to will it into existence, through the strength of their desire and their vibrational alignment.

But that very teaching **makes most people go passive**, waiting for life/the universe/God (use whatever label works for you) to show up and hand them what they desire.

They don't realize (because the teaching doesn't make it clear) that taking action in the right way, in alignment with your dreams and desires, is a critical element in actually getting what you want. Sitting there passively won't do it. The magic lies in the incredible power of your thoughts and desires combined with the awesome power to actually go and create.

But as time passes and those dreams and desires don't come into your reality, most people, whether they want to admit it or not, lose faith and eventually give up.

So many people now feel stuck, knowing that traditional goal setting hasn't worked for them, and neither has the more new age "law of attraction" approach.

They then feel that nothing will work for them, that their dreams are merely fantasies, and that they need to get realistic and make do with the life that they currently have.

It is an awful tragedy that through bad teaching, so much life is wasted, so many feel hopeless and that their dreams are out of reach.

When nothing could be further from the truth.

Success, as both Stephen and Andy told me separately, **is a process**. It is a matter of doing the right things in the right order.

It doesn't matter whether you do the right things in the right order consciously or unconsciously, by accident or on purpose.

Do it right and you will get what you desire. _Don't, and you won't_.

Some people do those things by default and most of the world calls them "lucky." But luck has nothing to do with it.

DESIGNING AND CREATING YOUR IDEAL LIFE

After design comes creation.

– STEPHEN HEDGER

I'm going to show you the step-by-step guide to creating your life by design – the process by which you get what you want in your life.

What I'm showing you is natural goal setting.

It is the way we were designed to get what we want in life. The most powerful truth I came to understand about this process was that it was how I had achieved the key things in my life already, I simply hadn't realized that.

Before I go through the steps, I first want you to understand a few things so that you get the most out of this section.

First, it is essential that you give yourself complete freedom to express what you truly desire. This is not about what you should want, not about what others think you should want; this isn't about keeping your real desires hidden away through any kind of fear or embarrassment about what others might think if they saw them.

If you don't give yourself complete freedom you will fall into the trap of using this process to **create a new and different version of what you don't want**. That isn't what you're here for. You unlock your ability to make truly astonishing things happen when you give yourself this complete freedom.

Second, and very, very importantly, completely let go of any sense of what's "realistic" for you.

Being "realistic" is a trap set by your ego to keep you stuck where you are, never really making progress. The truth is that none us have truly scratched the surface of our potential; none of us really understand what's realistic for us. And the ones that achieve massive success are really those who haven't given themselves the same constraints that 99% of people place *on themselves*.

As Steve Jobs so wisely said (slow down and consider the truth of what's being said here), "*The ones who are crazy enough to think they can change the world, are the ones who do.*"

So, make sure you've slowed down enough to understand the importance of what Steve Jobs said. He didn't say the ones who are *talented enough or clever enough, or lucky enough*, or with rich family and friends, with incredible academic success, or with great riches. He said it is the ones who think (know) they can change the world.

So, now for the sake of the dream life you can currently conceive of and the far, far, far more astonishing one that's actually available for you, let go of any sense of being realistic.

If the dream that inspires you is to build the next Amazon, go with that. If it is to go into space, go with that. Anytime you feel your ego pulling you back into being realistic, recognize that you are simply putting a lid, a restriction, on the amount of good you can receive through this process. Your life is too important and too precious for that.

Third, I want you to forget about goal setting. We are instead <u>designing</u> your dream life.

Goal setting is pain and hard work and playing small. Life designing is daydreaming about how wonderful to make your life. This is about enjoying and soaking in the most wonderful amazing vision for your life. It is about enjoying the truth that everything you dream of is possible for you.

It is about allowing your natural creation mechanism to breath once again, as it did when you were a child. To simply enjoy daydreaming about all the incredible possibilities for your life and choosing which ones to turn into reality.

What we're doing here isn't painful, isn't difficult, and isn't hard work. It's reconnecting you with your incredible creative power while you imagine your most incredible life.

OK, let's get started.

Step 1: Creating Your Desire List

The first thing we're going to do is actually work out what you really want. This may sound obvious but 99% of people really have absolutely no idea of what they want. They only have either a very vague idea of what they want (which doesn't help you) or they have a clear idea of what they don't want – they want to be out of debt, they want to lose weight, they want to quit their job etc. That isn't creation (your natural state).

The best way I know how to do this in on an Excel spreadsheet but by all means use a pen and paper or anything else that you feel is right for you. If you want to download the spreadsheet I used for this, go to www.unstoppableselfconfidence.com/bookbonuses to download the exact template I used.

So, the first step is to create a list of all your desires, everything you want in your life. Remember the guidelines I've given you in this section about giving yourself complete freedom. Write down everything that you desire. Write down as many things as you'd like.

Here are some things for you to consider as you do this:

- What would your perfect relationship look like?
- What would your ideal partner (or partners! – remember, no constraints) be like?
- What kind of place or places would you like to live?
- What would your dream home (or homes) be like?
- What kind of work would you like to do that would fill you with joy each day?
- What personal qualities would you like to have (or have more of)?
- What would you like your sex life to be like? (I will keep saying this: no constraints!)
- What skills would you like to master?
- What hobbies or fun things would you like to have more of in your life?
- Where would you like to go on vacation? How much of your time would you like to spend on vacation? How many vacations would you like each year?
- What car or cars would you love to have?
- What experiences would you love to have?

- Which people would you love to meet, love to work with, love to become friends with?
- Would you like vibrant, perfect health and energy?
- What kind of adventures would you like to have? Who would you like to have them with?
- What feelings would you like more of in your life?
- What kind of friends/social life/business contacts, etc. would you like to have in your life?
- What kind of help and support from others (paid or unpaid) would you like to have in your life?
- How would you like to spend your time if money was not a consideration?
- What would your dream life be like day to day, week to week, month to month, etc.?
- What are the things that you treat yourself with occasionally that you like more of in your life?

Give yourself as much time as you want or need on this. There is no rush; you don't need to do that anymore.

Can you start to see how getting specific about what you do want, instead of being vague and abstract about it, helps show your subconscious mind what to go out and actually get for you?

How by knowing specifically, clearly, and in detail what you want means that your incredible supercomputer can start filtering in and out of your conscious awareness all the people, situations, and circumstances that are exactly what you need to create those desires in your reality? There is incredible power in being specific.

Then, when you're ready, next to each desire give it a score based on how much you desire it. If you literally cannot imagine your life without it, rank it as 100%; 90%–100% means it is massively important to you; 80% means you really want it; and then 70% and below are the things that you'd love to have, things that would be great, but you feel less strongly about.

Don't overthink this part.

The trick here is to tune in to and listen to your <u>feelings</u>. Go with what <u>feels right</u> rather than what you think is right. Less thinking and more feelings will serve you well here. Your feelings are what you really want; your thoughts can get messed up by your ego.

Don't focus on whether you get it absolutely right – this isn't a test. You can always go back and change it whenever it feels right to do so. It's natural to do so.

Then put your desires in order, with the ones with the highest score in at the top. You're making clear to your subconscious mind through this process which desires you have the strongest emotional connection with.

Remember that **words are not our natural language** for communicating with our subconscious minds; **our feelings are**. Words are merely symbols to communicate those feelings. But one of the most important things you need to do to get your desires is communicate them accurately to your subconscious mind. And that means using your feelings **NOT your words**.

Forging that emotional connection with your desires is critical. The stronger your emotional connection, the more power you give to your subconscious mind to go and create in your life.

The way you do this is to get down on paper **the reason that you want this.** Again remember, this isn't a test. Only you decide what's right and wrong here. But allow yourself a little time to consider why you want this desire.

The clearer and more specific you can be, the better. The more you communicate to your subconscious mind the reasons you want each desire, the more power you give it to go and create it for you. The more emotion and feelings you connect to those reasons, the better.

The key here is to avoid simply saying "in order to be happy." I get that this is the underlying reason to do anything, but what you're searching for here is the reason before that. So, for example, a number of my reasons were things like:

- to be and express who I really am;
- to fulfill my true potential;
- to live life on my terms, not the life others want for me; and
- to live my life with the handbrake off.

The key here is that you make sure that the desires you've listed are really yours – not the desires that your friends, your parents, your teachers, your partner, those on social media, etc. think you should want. <u>But those that you really want</u>.

This is about going after the things that will truly, sincerely, make you the happiest, most fulfilled, most joyous that you could possibly be. You won't and can't reach that point if you are going after someone else's desires.

When I was going through this process, Stephen used to regularly challenge me to check that my designs were really my own. I ended up realizing that a number of the designs I put down were still "shoulds" rather than my real desires. Or they were limited visions of what I felt was "realistic"; or I hadn't put things on the list because, while I really wanted them, I was concerned that they would seem silly or embarrassing in some way.

Stephen was constantly challenging me to make sure I wasn't still holding back; that holding back was just another way my ego would put limits on my life. As Stephen said, this was the time to truly "let it rip."

So that's why you don't need to rush this process. The key is to find your authentic desires and simply follow the process.

I had about 80 things on my list when I first did this; 10 of which were 100% must haves; another 15–20 of which were in the 90%+ range; another 10–15 which were in the 70%–90% range. This isn't a target but the only guidance I'd give is to be focused around what you put in the 100% category. If you put everything in there, you're making your life more difficult.

Step 2: Creating Your Detailed Designs

One of the most famous quotes in personal development and success teaching is by Napoleon Hill which says:

"What the mind can conceive and believe it can achieve."

Andy taught me that this quote was so **nearly right**, so nearly transformative, but a couple of key things dissolved its incredible power for 99% of people. And that's why this next stage of the process is so important.

I've spoken earlier in the book about the problems with the word "believe," that it is weakness disguised as strength. It is doubt disguised as certainty. Well, the problem is that most success teaching gets people to focus on "believing they can." And so, without realizing it they are actually creating more doubt, more weakness, in their desires.

What they don't focus enough on is *knowing they can* and *conceiving their desire as real.*

Think of all the things you achieve day to day in your life right now: at home, in your job, with friends, holidays, trips to the shops. How many of those do you *believe* you can do?

How many of them do you simply *know you can do?*

When you slow down and think about it, how many of those things are in your mind, essentially complete, you just need to go and actually do them?

You have already *conceived* them in your mind as complete, done.

And so they happen, without strain, stress, or effort. You simply get on with making them your reality. You create (not achieve) them in your reality.

The same process is true for your big dreams and desires. It's just that most success teaching makes it somehow different, more difficult, and more complicated than the way you already actively create your life right now.

What Andy taught me and what transformed my ability to create my life by design is that this quote would be better worded as:

"What the mind can conceive and know, it can create."

Can you see, and, more importantly, can you feel how these slight changes to this great quote, these small but crucial changes in understanding about the meaning of the words, **transform its power**?

To conceive means to imagine your desire vividly, in full blown HD, in full detail; to see it as done and all the wonderful benefits and feelings it will give you as having already happened.

Knowing is not belief. Belief equals doubt. Knowing means no doubt, that ALL doubt is removed.

And then you simply go and create that dream, desire, or outcome in your reality, just like *you already do* with so much that you already have in your life.

That's a crucial point to understand so I want to ensure you don't miss it. *You already create your life by design, you simply do it unconsciously and far too often for things that you don't want or for things that you think you should want.*

That's why when you "expect" (which is really a different way of saying "know") bad things to happen, they often do. You are using this process brilliantly to create bad stuff.

Now I'm showing you how to use this to create the good stuff.

So, the next stage is to create your detailed designs, taking each of the key items on your desire list and working them up into fully detailed designs.

This is probably my favorite part of the whole process. It's where you can really dream about your life in incredibly rich detail. It's where you get to glimpse just how astonishing, incredible, and amazing your life can really be.

What you do here is take one thing from your desires list (and I recommend you take the item that matters to you the most) and then you create a detailed, vibrant, vivid picture in your mind of what your life looks like, what your life feels like, how you feel now that your desire has become part of your reality.

What's crucial here is that you write/create/feel this from the perspective of *your desire having already happened*.

Not will happen, not is happening, **but has already happened** and has been part of your reality for a period of time.

There are lots of different ways to do this. I use an app called Evernote to write out my designs so I can play with, refine, update, and simply read my designs on my desktop, phone, or iPad.

You may feel more comfortable using a mind map or a dream board or some other way. Use whichever method feels right for you.

The key is to take your time and build out the full, detailed, vivid, high-definition picture of just how wonderful your life is now that this design has become part of your reality. See and describe all the benefits to your life; see how it helped you on your journey to becoming the person you want to be and living the life you want to live.

See and feel how it benefitted not just you but all those you care about and all those around you. See how the completion of this design had benefits and opened doors to you completing other designs.

See how it all just happened naturally and fell into place for you, how having your design as part of your life feels completely normal and natural for you, familiar to you.

CREATE YOUR ANCHOR THOUGHT

I start off by coming up with what I call an "anchor thought" for each design. It is a picture in my mind of the image that most powerfully evokes the essence of what that design means for my life. And I find that once I have landed that anchor thought for each design, everything flows very naturally from there.

So, for example, one of my designs at the end of my divorce was buying my ex-wife out of her share of the house. This mattered a great deal to me. I wanted my daughters to keep the home they knew, the bedrooms that they were familiar with. In a time of great upheaval in their lives I wanted to give them as much stability as possible.

My anchor thought was me receiving the phone call from my lawyer telling me that the buy-out was complete. I was looking out of the window in my study to see my beautiful daughters, on a wonderful sunny day, bouncing on the trampoline in our back garden, happy and at peace, safe in their home, secure knowing that they didn't have to move. I remember seeing the peace and joy in their faces and they were playing; I remember feeling the joy and happiness of knowing that the buy-out was complete. I remember the happiness on the girls' faces when I told them that it was all OK, that it was done.

I remember having a beer in the garden with the girls playing around me, just closing my eyes and feeling the incredible, immense gratitude I had for the fact that this design had manifested. I remember feeling incredible realizing that if I could manifest this, then of course I could manifest my other designs as well. I remember the wonderful feeling of possibility that washed over me seeing that truth.

Well, that's **exactly** how it happened.

After I have landed my anchor thought, I go through and describe (in as much detail as feels right) how my life feels <u>having had</u> this design come into reality; how I feel now that this design being real has become part of my life.

You can do this in pictures or words but the key is that you turn up the volume of all the good feelings that having this design would bring to your life. Just keep writing or creating pictures that evoke as much great emotion in you as possible. Feel those feelings, soak in them, enjoy them.

SEE ALL THE WAYS IT COULD HAPPEN

After you've described your life and your feelings after the design has happened, the next stage is to feed your subconscious mind, with all of the ways this design could happen.

I want to be really clear here. This is not looking to define how your design **definitely will happen**, just the ways you can imagine **that it <u>could</u> happen**.

What you're doing here is feeding your subconscious mind, your incredible creation machine, with lots of data about the possible ways to make this desire, your design, come into your reality.

So, for example, with the design about buying my ex out of her share of the house, I saw lots of possible ways that could happen including:

- I was able to simply refinance the house to get the money needed.
- I saw that my other investments would provide me with enough funds.
- I saw that I could get a second charge loan on the house.
- I saw that I could start a business that would make me all the money I needed.
- I saw that I could pay her some of the money now and the rest of it over time.
- I saw that I could agree to different arrangements with my ex-wife, ones that would suit us both that allowed me to pay her over time. (I didn't know what these were, that was for my subconscious mind to figure out.)
- I saw that through a combination of personal loans, refinance, and my monthly income I could likely get most, if not all, of the money I needed and the rest would be a small balance over time.

There were many more besides but the point is that I was feeding my mind possibilities.

This is what the 1% do naturally and often without even realizing they're doing it. For 99% of people, the very second they dream of creating something in their lives, they allow their minds to instantly fill up with a laundry list of doubts, of ways that it won't happen, of ways that it would be hard, difficult, and so on.

Without even realizing it, they instantly sabotage their ability to create what they want by filling their subconscious minds with all the ways in which their designs _couldn't happen or won't happen_.

They fill their minds with pitfalls and consequences. So guess what their brilliant subconscious mind goes and finds? All kinds of miraculous, unbelievable ways that their designs get blocked, don't happen, cause problems, etc.

What I'm showing you here is how to communicate with your subconscious mind so that you get what you do want (which is what the 1% do on autopilot) instead of what you don't want (which is what the 99% do on autopilot).

Can you see that both the 1% and the 99% use the exact same process? It's just that the 99% use it to create bad stuff and the 1% use it to create what they desire.

All of us are naturally incredible creators. That isn't in doubt. It's just about consciously directing this incredible power so that you get what you want on demand instead of what you don't want by accident.

So for each of your designs, fill your mind with all the possibilities, all the possible ways that it could happen. You are literally programming a supercomputer to go to work for you here. Just consider each possible way, allow yourself to see how that way could deliver exactly what you need and would work out for the best for you.

You can then leave it up to your incredible subconscious mind to figure out (using all of that wonderful data you've just given it) the very best path to making your design a reality.

Step 3: Seeing it as Already Complete

Let me explain a little bit of what we're doing in this stage of the process and why, because I want you to understand the power of what you're doing here.

To bring any design into reality, to have it happen in your life, you need to know what you truly want; you need to create an emotional connection with that design by understanding how amazing it will make you feel when you have it in your life and you need to **see it in your mind as done, compete. You need to see it as having already happened in your mind**.

This matters, big time.

You see, your ego is hardwired to resist what is unfamiliar and to return to what is familiar.

Let me say that again because this is critical.

Your ego is hardwired to resist what is unfamiliar and to return to what is familiar.

What that means is that as you step forward towards your goals, towards your dream life, you are stepping into a life that is unfamiliar. If, as you read those words, you felt a little pang of fear or doubt then congratulations for proving my point perfectly. That was your ego poking you.

Your ego hates unfamiliar and so it throws all kinds of roadblocks, obstacles, bad feelings, fears, doubts, distractions your way – anything at all to stop you from moving from the familiar to the unfamiliar. Your ego's job is to keep you safe right where you are in the place, situation, or circumstance that you have previously experienced (and therefore survived).

It doesn't matter how good or shitty your current situation is – the fact that it's familiar is what matters to your ego.

The path to getting what you want is so much about simply getting out of your own way, about getting past these obstacles, fears, and doubts that your ego will throw at you. To do that, you need to show your ego, in a way that it understands, that the reality you're creating is familiar and safe.

This is why Stephen always told me that changing is easy **once people feel safe to change.**

You do this by going forward in time in your mind and experiencing your life with that desire having become part of your reality already. You daydream (remember as you did as a child) of how incredible you feel, now that you have that desire in your life, as a natural, normal, comfortable and completely wonderful part of your reality.

You're seeing it in your mind as having already happened.

It doesn't matter if (in your mind as you imagine it) it's just happened or happened a few weeks ago, a few days ago, or a few years ago. Just that it has already happened.

Here's the second part of this that makes all the difference. As you go forward in time in your mind and experience this, you will fill yourself up with all the incredible, wonderful feelings of gratitude that you have for having this in your life now. You soak in it.

Remember Andy's revision of that Napoleon Hill quote: "What your mind can conceive and know, it can create."

What we're doing here is moving you from belief (weak) to know (certain): by creating your designs in detail; by seeing all the incredible, wonderful benefits and feelings created by having design in your life; by filling your mind with all the possible ways it could happen, you are dissolving all the doubts that sabotage 99% of people as they go after their dreams.

By seeing it as done you are allowing your ego to see ahead of time, the life you are moving towards as familiar instead of unfamiliar.

By staying with your design and imagining it as having happened in your mind, you are conceiving it in detail, so your subconscious mind knows exactly what it needs to create for you and all the possible ways it can do it.

The critical point is that you stay imagining your design until in your mind it is done, complete, has happened. This is how you remove all doubt (the dream killer).

Remember, the key to getting exactly what you want isn't positive thinking, it is the removal of doubt.

Because this has become real in your mind, you reach the crucial tipping point, the point at which you're attached to your desires happening but at the same time relaxed and detached because in your mind it has already happened.

That combination of attached and yet detached at the same time (because you know it is certain) is the point at which you convert your designs from desires and possibilities into probabilities.

That is the point when you have given your mind everything you need to go and create what you desire.

You repeat that process with each of your designs.

Remember that these are your designs. You can change them, update them, modify them, delete them, and write new ones any time you like.

Step 4: After Design Comes Creation

The next stage is when you simply go out and start bringing your dreams into your reality. This isn't hard work. This is the most fun and joy you can have, creating your very best life with all the wonderful feelings that will bring.

This is you creating your reality just like you did when you were a child. You already know it is certain; you know you have nothing to fear. This is play.

As you start creating, be aware of your ego, still rearing up, still looking to sabotage your efforts with fears and doubts and distractions. Each time, remember not to fight or resist your ego. Instead to just still your mind, slow down, and bring in your 15 seconds of positive thought and get back in control of your mind.

Become the observer of your thoughts, separate from them. Look at them, consider them for value, and realize the truth: that all of them are tricks being played by your ego to keep you stuck.

Your ego will come up with a new trick when you begin bringing your designs into reality. It will try to make you feel overwhelmed and try to make you feel like creation is hard work. But in fact, bringing your designs into reality is just playing like you did when you were a child.

When you are creating the life you desire, don't focus on all the things you have to do to create it.

That takes something you love (your dream life) and turns it into hard work, which is pretty much the fastest way to destroy your progress.

Instead, still your mind, accept that everything that needs to get done will get done at the right time in the right way. Maybe not to the deadlines you originally thought or that others expect. But they will get done when the time is right.

How do I know this? Well, despite all the feelings of overwhelm in the past, you're still here, you've made it to today, so everything necessary for that to happen **has happened**.

Next, once you have calmed your mind, allow yourself to daydream, to see your dream life as already done, already created. See it as complete. Enjoy the feeling of it being done.

See and feel all the benefits to you and those you love from having created this life. Feel how amazing you feel.

Then focus on the next step you have to take to create that life and ONLY on that step.

Do whatever you need to do to complete it. Go about it in a workmanlike way until it is done. Don't try to start five other things or five other options. Just the next step and nothing more.

Then rinse and repeat, focusing on the amazing feelings you will have and the next step right in front of you.

Imagine if you did this for one year, three years, five years, or even the rest of your life?

Then instead of feeling overwhelmed with bad feelings, you would create amazing feelings and continual progress.

Just imagine how quickly you could create the life of your dreams then?

RECAP OF THE LIFE DESIGN PROCESS

1. Create your list of your life desires.

2. Score each desire with a percentage of how important it is to you.

3. Rank your desires in order of importance.

4. Work out why you want it, to make sure you really do want it and not just think you should want it.

5. Start creating your detailed designs.

6. Find your anchor thought for each one.

7. See all the ways it could happen – not definitely will happen, just could.

8. In your mind, go forward in time and see your designs as done, complete, as having already happened.

9. Having this design as part of your life, feel the incredible feelings, the incredible sense of gratitude.

10. Keep going until you have removed all doubts.

11. Go and create and keep going UNTIL your designs have become your reality. Focus on taking the next step and only the next step. Then the next, then the next.

THINGS TO CONSIDER

- Do you know what you want? Slow down and think about this. Do you know clearly and in detail what you want, or only vaguely? Do you only know what you don't want or what you should want?

- Do you know what your dream life looks like in detail?

- Imagine what your dream life would look like, without any constraints or restrictions **_at all._** No financial restrictions, no need to be realistic, no restrictions about what others might think. This is complete freedom to daydream.

- Can you see why mainstream goal setting actually kills your dreams dead, by getting you to be realistic and making your dream hard work?

- Can you see the difference in power between setting goals and designing your life?

- Consider that any "shoulds" will sabotage your success.

- Can you see that you create your dreams – you do not attract them.

HOW TO LIVE LIFE ON PURPOSE

> **The purpose of life is to find your gift. The meaning of life is to give it away.**
>
> DAVID VISCOTT

Life falls into place when you live your life "on purpose."

When you live your life in complete alignment with what inspires you, with what fills you up instead of emptying you out.

When you live fully expressing all of your gifts and talents in alignment and pursuit of that which gives you your greatest inspiration.

Once you know your purpose, it becomes the "magnetic north" of your life alongside your values. Distractions, negative thinking, lack of confidence, any obstacles at all, simply fall away because you're so inspired by what you are doing. You move past those things because they are getting in the way of something you **feel compelled to do**.

All your choices, all your actions, all your decisions naturally and without effort, line up along the right path that has always been there, waiting for you to follow it.

And there is a structured way for you (yes, you!) to find your mission.

You simply need to give this question to your subconscious mind, that part of your mind that is almost infinitely powerful. It already knows what your mission is, what your life purpose is, so you can relax and enjoy this process.

The answer already exists; all we're doing is clearing away the layers of dust that are keeping it hidden.

But first I want to give you a personal story to explain why finding your purpose is so important and so powerful.

For much of my adult life, I had, by most traditional standards, done "pretty well." I was pretty wealthy; I was pretty successful in my career; I had done pretty well through investing in real estate; I had done pretty well in my love life; I lived in a pretty nice home. Pretty much you name it and I was doing "pretty well."

Now maybe that all sounds good. What's to complain about?

Well, here's the thing. I was frustrated, deeply frustrated. Deep down I knew I was capable of much, much more. Of a much, much better, much, much more fulfilling life.

I didn't want the story of my life to be "pretty good." I wanted it to be the very best it could possibly be.

I made numerous attempts at creating that life. I dabbled in countless investments; I started a number of different businesses. They all started "pretty well" (are you seeing the theme here?) but somehow, in some way, all just kind of fizzled out.

I remember on my fortieth birthday getting a video message from two really great friends. I love them both dearly and they both want nothing but the very best for me. They were (with love and affection) jabbing at me like male friends do on these occasions.

In the video they went through a list of "accomplishments" in my life and at the end of each one asked, "Where's that now?" noting how each accomplishment had fallen away; that what had been built up had fallen down.

And what I knew, that they couldn't have known, was that the same was true of my marriage. Another thing that at one time had been "pretty good" was now in pieces.

Each of these "pretty good" things were built up and fell away because I was motivated by them, I wasn't inspired by them. Whenever an obstacle hit, it depleted my energy. Each step forward required a huge amount of effort, stress, and strain, where I reminded myself how much I wanted this, how if I wanted this, I simply had no choice but to buckle down and work hard for it. That I needed to hustle.

But the truth was, it was exhausting me. None of the things I was doing were inspiring me. Each step forward drained my energy instead of adding to it.

SIDE NOTE

One point about money here. The trap that many people fall into is thinking that their purpose is "to get rich" or "to be financially free." This is a mistake. There's absolutely nothing wrong at all with wanting wealth. Far from it. But your fast path to wealth comes from finding your true purpose first.

Despite what you may think, you don't actually want money per se. You want what money will do for you.

Your purpose is what you would do even if you had billions in the bank and never, ever needed to work again. It is about finding a central core to your life so that on the last day of your life you will be happy that yours was a life well lived.

MOTIVATION IS TEMPORARY, INSPIRATION LASTS FOREVER

And that's the problem with motivation: the world thinks it's something great (as I did too until Andy showed me how wrongheaded this way of thinking was), but in terms of achieving your important goals, the ones that really matter to you, it's terrible and destructive.

What I'm about to tell you goes completely against what almost the whole world BELIEVES to be true and so your ego is going to go into overdrive to get you to dismiss what I'm saying here.

Nearly the whole world talks about motivation, and yet 99% of people don't get what they want in life.

That's because motivation is actually pretty weak. It requires big effort and so ultimately works against you.

Let me explain.

When you are inspired, you no longer need motivation at all. In fact, it seems crazy.

When you really look at it, you realize that you only need motivation for things you don't really want to do (which should be your first indication that trying to get motivated works against you).

Whereas when you find your true purpose, your mission in life, you feel _**inspired**_. You just do whatever it takes to bring that dream into reality because you cannot imagine **not doing that**.

People need motivation when they "try" to do something that they don't really want to do. It can work for short periods of time, but it requires a lot of energy and constantly needs to be topped up.

Whereas you only really need to get inspired once. And when you do, you will have all the fuel you need to send you flying on your journey.

Lots of successful people use the word "motivation" when in fact they mean _**inspired**_. And so, through a small misinterpretation, huge problems are caused for 99% of people.

Show me anything truly great that anyone has done and I will show you someone inspired **not** motivated.

Steve Jobs, Elon Musk, Mark Zuckerberg, Marie Curie, Nelson Mandela, Oprah Winfrey, Winston Churchill, Jeff Bezos, Walt Disney, J.K.

Rowling, Thomas Edison, and countless others, famous and unknown, were all inspired. And as a result, they overcame incredible obstacles.

Needing motivation is a signpost telling you that you don't yet know what you truly want.

Find your inspiration, your purpose, and feel the difference it makes.

There is nothing more unstoppable than someone inspired.

When you're inspired each step forward, each stage, each thing you do doesn't deplete your energy. Inspiration is an essentially unlimited supply of energy.

Whereas motivation requires constant replenishment, constant effort.

That's why people who are inspired say that they've never really worked a day in their life despite working long hours and doing things that most people would find exhausting.

Can you see how critical being inspired is to the success of your journey? Can you see how finding your purpose unlocks your hidden reservoir of unlimited energy and persistence?

THE STRUCTURED PROCESS FOR DISCOVERING YOUR LIFE PURPOSE

We're here to put a dent in the universe.
Otherwise why else even be here?

– STEVE JOBS

As we go into this process, I'd like you to still your mind and relax. What we're doing here is communicating with your subconscious mind so that it gives you the perfect answer for you.

This process will work, but the more relaxed and open you are to it, the faster and more effective it will be.

Remember, you've come this far; you're reading this book because you're looking for answers. I absolutely want you to find your purpose and I'm showing the very best, proven way to do that. So just trust in this process and follow the steps outlined here.

Your future self will be incredibly grateful that you did.

For the next few minutes, I'd like you to see yourself in the future having found your purpose.

Imagine for a moment the feelings you will feel when you uncover your mission in life; the thing that your unique talents and experiences equip you perfectly for; the thing that you would love to do, no matter what, no matter the money you had in the bank; the calling that would add to every aspect and facet of your life, that would unlock the incredible, awesome potential within you.

Imagine in your mind the incredible excitement and passion, the incredible intoxicating sense of possibility you will feel once your subconscious mind has revealed your purpose to you.

See in your mind how obvious it was, how when it was revealed to you, you could hardly believe you hadn't already seen it, it was just so obvious, so clear, so right.

How finding your purpose was the start of an amazing transformation of your life; how so much simply fell into place after you discovered and then lived your purpose.

How finding your purpose unlocked you getting everything else you desired in your life, in your personal life, in your work life, in terms of wealth, in terms of lifestyle. Everything.

See how you couldn't out-give the universe, how with each interaction you gave incredible value to the world around you and those you love, and how you were rewarded with breathtaking abundance in every way that matters to you as a result. The more you gave the more you were rewarded.

See how your successes accumulated and how you helped others on their journey too.

See how, as Steve Jobs so wisely said, you couldn't see how all the dots joined up at the time but now looking back you can see how your life was actually falling perfectly into place. Every experience, every challenge, every difficult moment, all of it was giving you exactly what you needed to fulfill your purpose.

See how rewarding your day-to-day experience of life became as people you interacted with thanked you for the amazing things you did for them.

See how this was the starting point for your very best life, the life you dreamed of, living as the very best version of you each and every day.

So let's get started.

Step 1: Defining What Your Purpose Looks Like

The first step in this process is to come up with a list of things that you know you want your life purpose to look like and give you. What you're doing here is setting out the qualities, the features, the details of what would make a purpose perfect for you.

This isn't trying to write down what your life purpose is. It is about how it will make you feel, what it would make your life like, the kind of set-up and experiences your perfect purpose would give you, and the ways it would allow you to live. It's the kinds of things you want to do with your life.

What we're doing here is feeding your subconscious mind with all the data it needs to discover your purpose and feed it back to you.

The better data you give it, which is defined by the degree of emotion each point creates within you, the quicker it can go to work for you figuring this all out.

As with the previous chapter, do not put any limits or constraints on yourself or your thinking here.

Remember, this is about discovering your perfect purpose, which gives you your dream life on your terms. So don't hold back. Really let it rip with this.

You can do this with a pen and paper, with a list or a mind map.

I found the most effective way for me was with a mind map but choose what feels right for you.

If you go to www.unstoppableselfconfidence.com/bookbonuses, you can download an example mind map that you can use or adjust to suit you.

Start to write out a list of things that you want your dream purpose to look like and give you. Think about what you want to do with your life; think about what it would look like and feel like to you.

Here's some of the things I wrote down for me:

- To do something where I teach and become a master of all the skills I most want to learn and develop.
- To build a business that gives me complete freedom to be around for my daughters, so I'm around as they grow up.
- To do something I am uniquely equipped to do.
- To have fun doing something that I love.
- To do something where I crack the system for a problem that makes it easy for others to follow the path.
- To leave a legacy.
- To be able to work when I want, as much as I want, from wherever I want.
- To do something that fills me with energy so that I never work another day in my life.
- To have the platform to inspire lots of people to live their best lives.
- To create something that would last a lifetime and would grow throughout my lifetime.
- To write a book.
- To work with people who would inspire me to ever-greater heights.

- To create a business that gave me all the income I ever needed to create an incredible life for me, my daughters, and those closest to me.
- To do something that gave me the opportunity to travel around the world and be paid to do it.
- To do something that built and developed my mindset each and every day.
- To do something where my day-to-day work would support me becoming the very best version of me each and every day.
- To create a business where I didn't need lots of start-up capital or need to loads of employees to run. A simple, low hassle, highly profitable, and cashflow positive business.
- To create a business that makes me a better parent.
- To create a business that creates a self-sustaining and abundant revenue stream that constantly increases.
- To create a fortune that allows me to live life on my terms.
- To do something that completely aligns with and supports my values.

By having this list, the list of things that would make my life **_exactly_** as I wanted it to be, I set the framework for what my purpose would look like. I knew that my purpose would fit all of these things.

Your list may look very similar or completely different. I have only put my list down here to give you some inspiration about the kinds of things you may wish to consider.

Notice (**feel**) that I didn't hold back or put any constraints on myself. Notice (**feel**) how there is no need for motivation in any of this. Notice (**feel**) how inspired I am by each and every one of those points.

Notice (**feel**) how I am creating something that adds to the world with every interaction and transaction, and this provides the platform for my best life on my terms.

So, take a little bit of time here. Go and create the list that's right for you.

Download the free mind map to use for this and fill in the list of things that are right for you.

Here's the link again: *www.unstoppableselfconfidence.com/bookbonuses.*

You can't get this wrong. The only way you "get it wrong" is by not doing it.

Don't move on to the next stage until you've done this.

Step 2: Consider Each Point in Turn: What Would Fit Your List?

The next stage after you've completed your list is to consider each point in turn, and think about what would fit that point plus all the others on your list.

This is why I prefer to do this on a mind map – so I could mentally cycle around each point and ask my subconscious mind, "What would fit all the things on my list?"

What you're doing here is setting your subconscious mind to work for you, on answering this question.

So, I picked my first point which was "to do something where I teach and become a master of all the skills I most want to learn and develop." I just pondered: What would fit that desire?

I filled my subconscious mind with data about what could (not definitely would) fit all the desires for my purpose that I had listed out. I didn't try to instantly find a silver bullet answer. I just considered the possibilities.

I waited to see if an answer was coming. I relaxed if it didn't and went on to consider the next point. This was "to build a business that gives me complete freedom to be around for my daughters, so I'm around as they grow up."

So I considered the skills I most wanted to learn and whether I could build a business teaching those skills that would allow me to be around for my daughters. What would that business look like?

I then considered the next point which was "to do something I am uniquely equipped to do." I thought about my skill set. I didn't give in to bullshit false modesty here. I allowed myself to consider all the things that I knew I was good at, all the natural talents I knew I had, all the things that people had repeatedly told me I was good at.

For every point in turn, I considered the possibilities and options. I went around my mind map filling my subconscious mind with all the data it needed.

Most importantly, I <u>trusted</u> that my subconscious mind, the incredible, breathtakingly powerful supercomputer between my ears would give me the answer <u>at the right time and in the right way</u>.

Step 3: Allow the Answer to Emerge: Don't Force It

The trick is not to force the answer but to *allow* the answer to emerge.

This process can take minutes, hours, days, weeks, or sometimes even months. But don't fear that. Instead, enjoy the process of discovering your calling. Be excited about the fact that the answer is coming. Embrace it.

Because getting the answer to your mission in life is the most incredible, empowering, life-changing work you can do.

Trust that your subconscious mind is working on the answer – because it is. The answer will emerge if you trust that it will. If you doubt that it will, that will become true just as easily.

Then at the right time in the right way, when you've considered this question and given your subconscious mind the chance to find the answer for you, the answer will emerge. You may be taking a walk, in the shower, at the gym, just going about your day, and suddenly the answer will just appear in your mind.

You will know, without any question or doubt when it happens. <u>You will likely be shocked at just how obvious the answer is</u>, how it was hidden in plain sight.

How in reality you always knew this was your purpose, but had somehow never quite consciously landed it. That's because the answer was always there in your brilliant subconscious mind. You just have to learn how to communicate with it in the right way.

So many people who have used this process have said that their purpose was staring them in the face the whole time; that it was right there in front of them the whole time; that they were stressing and straining trying to figure out what it was.

I found my purpose through exactly this process. Let me explain a little more about how it happened.

It actually took me around three months for it to finally hit me, but when it did, it was like a bright light just turned on in my mind.

I created the list I wrote out earlier. I went through each point as I described. I went around them many times just considering what my unique purpose could be. I felt stuck many times, feeling like the answer would never come. But I trusted that my subconscious mind would find the answer. I simply needed to trust the process.

Each day I spent a little time thinking about it. Each evening as I went to sleep, I asked my subconscious mind to give me the answer.

While all the points were really important to me, there were a few that really stuck out, ones that were like my anchor points if you like. These were: the desire to teach the skills that I most wanted to master, to do something that allowed me to earn a lot of money while being around for my daughters, and to have fun doing something that I love so that I never feel like I work another day in my life.

I was considering the point about the skills that I would most like to learn, and had been for a few days.

Then one day, I was in a taxi on the way to the airport. The question was just working its way through my subconscious mind; I was only vaguely aware that I was thinking about it at all. I remember the taxi was just pulling into the drop off area for the terminal when suddenly it just hit me with a bang. As I said, it was like someone switched on every light bulb in the world all at once. It was like a physical jolt of energy.

I remember just saying, "That's it! Of course. OF FUCKING COURSE!"

I would teach the world how to be confident: not pretend confident, not arrogant frat boy confident, not some bullshit "tell yourself you're really great" or fake it until you make it confident, not confident that lasts for a short time and then fades away.

Real, true, natural, indestructible, bulletproof, unshakable, lifelong, lasting confidence that unlocks everything you ever wanted in life.

I went back through my list.

Was this something I would happily spend the rest of my life learning, mastering, and teaching? For sure it was.

Was it something I was uniquely equipped to do? Yes, I had been on an incredible journey around reconnecting with my own natural confidence and I had learned from the very best teachers in the world. <u>I knew the path and had walked the path</u>.

Many people had previously told me that I had an incredible talent for taking things that seemed difficult or complicated and making them easy and accessible – that I knew how to crack the system to make what others make hard, seem easy.

Was it something that I would have fun doing and never feel like I worked another day in my life? Yes!

Was it something that I could create a self-sustaining and abundant revenue stream from? Yes!

Would it give me a platform to inspire others? Without question. As I sat in the airport reading back over my list on my phone, I realized that the answer my subconscious mind had given me fitted every single point I wrote down. **EVERY SINGLE ONE.**

I felt an incredible surge of excitement as I realized I had just taken a huge step towards my very best life.

UNLOCKING YOUR GREATNESS

The difference between great people and everyone else is that great people create their lives actively, while everyone else is created by their lives, passively waiting to see where life takes them next.

– MICHAEL GERBER

Unlocking all of your incredible potential – living your very best life – requires you living your life on purpose.

You unleash the full spectrum and the full power of your talents when you find your purpose and live your purpose. It is one of the master keys to living a life that few can even conceive.

So consider, before you move on, whether you wish to discover and unleash the greatness within you.

On the day you die, how much of your potential will you have left untouched?

How much of what you could achieve will you have done? How much of the incredible life you can create will you have lived?

Will you do all the things you dream of doing? Will you become the person you dream of becoming?

Will you get the most you possibly can out of this life (the only one you KNOW for certain that you have)?

Or will you play it safe and settle for an average life like 99% of people? And be clear that to "settle" means to give up on your dreams, to let your talents and gifts wither and die.

Most people let the greatness within them, all the incredible talent and gifts they have been given, go to waste.

Most people give up on their dreams because they decide, without taking the steps that would create their dream life, that it is unrealistic.

Most people let bad programming, backwards teaching, and stifling social conditioning keep them stuck and playing small and making what only appears to be the safe choice – but without realizing that the safe choice is actually the riskiest choice there is, because it comes with the CERTAIN cost of never living life on your terms.

Everyone who is born, everyone who has ever lived, has greatness within them. And yes, that includes you.

The difference between the 1% who unleash that greatness and the 99% who waste it, is choice.

Choice is always the problem and the solution. If you choose (which means consistently act) to unleash **YOUR** greatness you **WILL** achieve it – and with it the life of your dreams.

But most people choose not to. Not because they cannot do it, but because they decide it isn't possible; because they decide to play it safe; because they decide they aren't worthy of being great; because they decide that isn't realistic.

You can choose to believe these lies that suffocate most of the world. Or you can choose to see the truth that your dream life is not only possible but probable if you take the right steps.

The question is not whether you have greatness within you. You do.

The question is whether you will decide to unleash it or waste it.

What choice will you make?

THINGS TO CONSIDER

- Can you see the incredible power of discovering your purpose and of living your life "on purpose"?

- Consider that finding your purpose is the key to unleashing the greatness that exists within you.

- Knowing your purpose alongside your values means that decision-making is easy. Each decision, each choice, either helps you on your incredible, inspiring journey or it distracts and takes you away from it.

- Can you see how the whole idea of motivation is a trap? That if you need motivation, you are doing something you should, something that drains your energy instead of filling it up.

- Consider that you now have a structured way of finding your purpose. Is there any reason not to go and discover your calling?

CHAPTER 17

UNLEASHING YOUR NATURAL ABUNDANCE

> Expect your every need to be met. Expect the answer to every problem. Expect abundance on every level.
>
> EILEEN CADDY

Do you expect abundance in your life?

This is one of the questions where it's important that you slow down and feel your answer rather than answering straightaway.

Because the answer you feel (rather than think) will go a long way to showing why you may not yet have seen the abundance in your life that you would like.

We love the idea of abundance, but deep down, hidden away, so many people don't really feel like they deserve abundance or that it's "realistic" for them.

What they don't realize is that it is only that feeling that is blocking them from accessing and seeing the abundance that is available for them right now and **staring them in the face**.

Because most people believe "lack" to be their underlying truth, they unconsciously program their subconscious minds to seek out lack.

Their subconscious mind dutifully and faithfully follows that command exactly. It <u>filters in</u> to their conscious awareness all the forms of lack and <u>filters out</u> the abundance that exists around them.

And so, *lack becomes their reality*.

Remember that we communicate with our subconscious minds (our incredible creation mechanism) through our feelings (our natural language) not our words which are mere symbols for those feelings. That's why if you say "I want to be a millionaire" it doesn't work. You instead need to communicate to your subconscious mind the incredible, wonderful, abundant feelings that you have from **already** (in your mind) being a millionaire.

Then it will seek out and find all kinds of incredible, unexpected, and frankly jaw-dropping ways that being a millionaire will happen for you.

The same is true for an answer to any problem, for the people who can help you, for the opportunities you would like. For anything at all. <u>There is no limit to this</u>.

It is all about what you consciously or unconsciously program your subconscious mind to filter in to and out of your consciousness.

Remember, you program your mind through your dominant thoughts.

This is one of the many reasons that controlling your mind and so being able to *direct and focus your thoughts and emotions* is so important.

Let me give you an example of this.

The way I first got to know Andy Shaw was through real estate investing. It had been something I had been interested in doing for some time, but I had never found a deal that made sense to me.

I thought the deals were no longer there. I "believed" that prices had risen too far and that I had "missed the boat" on property investing and it was too late – that all the good deals had already gone.

I searched and searched but concluded, with my lack mindset at the time, that there were no deals.

At the time, Andy hosted lunches for aspiring property investors at his home and I managed to get along to one. I remember Andy being asked about the current deals he was doing, and how many he was doing right now.

He said (from memory) that he had around 15 deals going through at that particular time and each would make him (at the point he bought them) between £10K and £20K each in cash.

I said to him, as did several others, that he must simply be lucky with the areas he was buying in because no such deals were available in our local areas.

Andy smiled and told us he would find a deal in each of our areas within five minutes.

He sat at his computer and logged onto the main property portal in the UK and asked me for my area.

Within three minutes he had found a deal that had been sitting there in plain sight, explained the reasons it was such a great deal, and then added a few simple tricks to make it even more lucrative.

The property in question was one I had looked at, evaluated, and dismissed already. It wasn't a new deal; it was one sitting there waiting to be snapped up.

The difference was that I had evaluated the deal with a _deprivation mindset_ and Andy had evaluated it with an _abundance mindset_.

I was assessing the deal, and my mind (unconsciously) was tuned to looking for what could go wrong, where I might lose money, and the risks and challenges that the deal may present me with.

Andy was assessing the deal with his mind (both consciously and unconsciously), seeing the abundance that was right there in front of both of us. He saw all that could go right, all the many different ways money could be made from the deal, all the ways it could be made as lucrative as possible.

Andy was tuned into abundance so he saw abundance where others saw lack; he saw abundance everywhere.

The facts weren't any different. It was the same property, the same price, the same possibilities, and the same risks.

From that one deal I directly made £20K and, overall, thanks to Andy's teaching, I probably made a little over £500K from property investing – all from being taught how to tune into the abundance that was always there but that I had tuned out.

DEPRIVATION THINKING VS. ABUNDANCE THINKING

We do not see things as they are, we see things as we are.

– ANAIS NIN

It is very, very easy to become a highly trained deprivation thinker. I say highly trained because your natural default is to think abundance.

So, despite what you may think, *a lot* of training and reprogramming is needed to switch your default away from your natural abundant thinking state that you had as a child into a state of deprivation and lack.

But that programming is exactly what we are bombarded with every day. Nearly all the training we receive as we grow up from well- (or badly-) intentioned teachers, social media, TV, parents, friends, and peers is focused on deprivation.

You may recall from an earlier chapter that I said *your default state is the state you're most often in*.

So, if you're progressively trained and programmed to see lack, then seeing lack instead of abundance will become your default state.

Through a subtle but important shift in your daily habits, you can rewire your brain, your mind, <u>to focus on and see abundance or lack just as easily</u>.

Watch enough TV focused on all the bad things, all the negativity and lack in the world (and excluding all the wonderful, beautiful, and abundant because good news is rarely deemed "newsworthy"), hear enough people with deprivation thinking talk about all the problems they face, see enough things on social media parading negativity, then soon enough our unguarded minds will be fully programmed to <u>filter in the appearance of lack and filter out the truth of the incredible abundance hiding in plain sight</u>.

Soon enough this becomes what we perceive to be the underlying "truth." And through our mind's cognitive bias, **we only see what we "know" to be true**.

Cognitive bias means that we only tend to see that which supports our belief systems and we tend to be blind to that which challenges them.

My cognitive bias (of deprivation and lack) with property deals at the time I met Andy was that the truth was that there were no good deals left. So, I was blind to the deals that were right in front of me.

Andy's cognitive bias of abundance <u>revealed the underlying truth</u> to him that deals were widely and easily available.

Primarily seeing deprivation and lack is the key way that 99% of people block the incredible abundance that surrounds them.

A REMINDER ABOUT MIND CONTROL

You may also recall from earlier in the book that I talked about the foundational importance of your ability to control your thoughts, about having the ability to think thoughts that help you instead of those that harm you.

Well, this is where "shit gets real."

Because it is only by having the ability to control your thoughts that you can tune into the abundance around you and *stay tuned into it.*

The negative noise, nonsense, and propaganda from the world isn't going away any time soon. Unless you have the ability to control your thinking, it can and will, subtly and without you noticing, start taking you away from the right ways of abundant thought into deprivation and lack thought.

You have two lines of defense and protection against deprivation thinking. The first is to continue to be conscious and to observe your thoughts. And the second is to choose your natural abundant thoughts **not the unnatural, programmed deprivation thoughts**.

I always keep a bit of my awareness focused on how I am thinking and feeling. I observe when I start to feel down, bad, or limited in any way.

The moment I feel myself drifting towards negativity or deprivation, it is a prompt to go and get back in control of my mind. I do this several times each day, whenever I feel I need to. Each time I do, I am amazed at how my day just gets easier, how problems resolve themselves (another form of abundance), and how unexpected good just flows into my life.

I am always surprised at how quickly and easily I return to my natural abundant state just by following this simple and easy practice.

On the rare occasions now where my ego briefly gets control, I realize that my day is much, much harder, problems just appear out of seemingly nowhere, and even previously resolved problems get unresolved.

HOW AND WHY MOST PEOPLE CREATE LACK

Most people struggle with the concept of abundance intellectually but more importantly _they struggle with it emotionally_.

They think it is unrealistic, hippie, new age bullshit.

They almost always react against *even the idea* of the world being full of abundance, of them being abundant beings, of the potential for their lives to be filled with abundance at every level.

Because accepting (or even just being open to) the truth of abundance means admitting your view of the world is wrong. And our egos absolutely hate us admitting we're wrong. Our egos prefer us to be "right" (locked into our existing views) rather than to be happy by being ready to be wrong and change. Because then we might and go and do something new.

But the problem with refusing to being open to being wrong is that it means all thinking has stopped. And so new possibilities, however much potential they hold, are easily dismissed.

HOW AND WHY MOST PEOPLE CREATE LACK

Let me show you just some of the ways that 99% of people create lack in their lives, how they take all the incredible abundance, possibility, and opportunity around them and shrink it into almost nothingness.

As you go through this section, slow down and consider the ways in which you have done the things I will describe. I know I have done all of them.

And remember, don't feel bad or judge yourself for having made these mistakes. There's no value in that for you and all you are interested in is what helps you.

But first of all, I want you to imagine for a second that you are in a massive room at the center of a huge factory and warehouse. There are conveyor belts – big, wide, free-flowing conveyor belts – channeling into that room (to you) whatever you need, on demand. No matter what you desire or what you ask for, those conveyor belts somehow always bring you something bigger and better.

Each conveyor belt represents a different type of supply (abundance): one for material wealth, one for love, one for great feelings, one for friendship, one for purpose, one for opportunity, one for health, one for solving problems.

There is a conveyor belt for every type of abundance imaginable, all directly channeling incredible good and abundance to you 24 hours a day, 7 days a week, 365 days a year.

There is no limit to the amount of good **you can receive**, but you can limit the amount of abundance that **actually reaches you**.

Each time, in each way, that you think the wrong way instead of the right way, I want you to imagine that you are blocking up those conveyor belts, impeding the flow of abundance and good into your life.

The more wrong ways that you think, the more you block up the flow. Each time you think the right way, you unblock it a little or a lot.

The issue is not the supply coming to you – it's you blocking up the conveyor belt that stops from it reaching you.

The single biggest block that we've already discussed is not knowing that abundance is the truth. That means that even when incredible abundance is right in front of you, flowing right past your face, you don't recognize it as abundance: you dismiss it as meant for someone else; you ignore it because you "know" that abundance isn't the truth, only deprivation and lack.

The second biggest block comes from your sense of "should." What I mean is that most people pre-judge that abundance *can only come* in the form that they have already decided it must look like. If something appears in their life that doesn't look *precisely as they've decided it should*, it is instantly dismissed. The abundance is ignored or dismissed. The conveyor belt is further blocked up, only allowing things into the room that come in that predetermined shape or form.

So, for example, you may have decided that one specific job is the perfect job for you. However, the truth is that you don't know and can't know everything about that job. So, it may be the perfect job for you **or it may not be**. But you may have already pictured in your mind how amazing the job will be, how great the people will be, how this job will be so different to the last one.

You have become attached to the outcome that you have decided is now the only right outcome.

Maybe a different job is actually perfect for you but just looks different from how it "should" look. Maybe the different job offers you opportunities for career progression, growth, pay, and benefits that are way, way, way beyond the job that you've targeted.

And so, you restrict the amount of abundance that you receive (not the amount that's available to you) by only allowing in abundance that looks the way you think it should.

The next major way most people block abundance is <u>through their self-imposed fears and limits</u>. They decide that certain things "aren't possible" for them, "won't happen" for them, "aren't realistic" for them. None of this is the truth, but it becomes their truth, directly as a result of them making that decision.

They see the world through the lens of what could go wrong, the downsides, the consequences, and the risks. As a result, all kinds of abundance, all kinds of opportunities, all kinds of joy and wonder are blocked, because they see the world through a deprivation lens.

They end up not grasping the abundance that they almost certainly know deep down is abundance because their fears and limits are in control of their mind.

They may have no more evidence that things could go wrong than that they could go right. But they fall for their ego's lies that where they currently are and what they currently know is safe and secure.

As a result, they **send back the opportunities to experience more**, to be more, to have more, to live more, because their focus is purely on the risks of taking action, never on the risks of standing still.

Our egos love us only looking at one side of the risk equation, never the full picture.

They ignore the incredible business or investment opportunity that's right in front of them because they decide it's too risky, and yet will not consider the risks to their life of never fulfilling their dreams, never having quite enough money to not live a highly restricted life, of never being able to live a life that lights them up.

They block opportunity after opportunity to approach that hot girl or guy that they really like because they think they're "out of their league." They don't go after their dreams because they've decided that it isn't meant to happen for them.

And so, the conveyor belt gets blocked up ever further.

The last way abundance gets block is through believing in luck. Luck is an entirely disempowering belief that says that the quality of your life and what happens to you is determined by fate, not by the choices, decisions, and actions that you take.

A belief in luck slowly kills off your incredible ability to create all the abundance that you desire, because it says that that life is something *that happens to you instead of by you*.

It causes you to sit passively, waiting for luck to be delivered to you, instead of you following your natural model of creating your life as you wish it to be. And if you have decided that **not only do you believe in luck but that you are unlucky**, then you have decided to make yourself helpless and entirely passive. You stop being part of the creation and management of your life. You become a victim of it. All through a false belief.

Because luck, at least in the way that 99% of people understand it, doesn't exist.

Stop and consider for a moment: Do you believe in luck?

Do you believe that the circumstances of your life are determined in ways big and small by the cards you have been dealt or the roll of the dice?

If so, why?

Do you really have any evidence that the quality of your life is determined by a force utterly outside of your control?

The problem with this way of thinking is that it makes you passive and weak. It says you're a victim of circumstance instead of the author of your story. It's says that there's no point is really trying anything, because you've decided that you're not a lucky person.

This is the perfect recipe for keeping you stuck, playing small, not looking to take the very steps that would make you what the world calls "lucky."

The 1% have simply learned to take action and think in ways that make them *appear lucky* compared to the 99%. But those actions and ways of thinking are yours to adopt any time you choose.

It simply means taking 100% responsibility for your life, seeing the open doors right in front of you and actually walking through them.

It means knowing what you truly want instead of just what you don't want or what you should want. It means taking steps each day towards becoming who you want to be and creating the life you want to live.

And it means focusing on thinking in the right ways so that there's no room to think in the ways that block your success and keep you stuck.

You need to take 100% responsibility for your life if you want to live it on your terms.

Luck, like confidence and success, is a choice even if nearly the whole world tells you otherwise.

The power lies within you, <u>not outside of you</u>.

Luck is simply seeing that truth and more importantly living that truth.

Can you see how each one of these layers of deprivation thinking, of the false limits that have been programmed into you, all work against you actually seeing and receiving the abundance that exists right there, right now in front of you?

Can you see and feel how you have limited your own abundance by thinking some or many of these lack thoughts?

Can you now see, when you look back on your life, how there was far more abundance waiting for you if only you reached out and grabbed it?

I very deliberately saved this chapter until later in the book, because I knew that it is only possible to grasp the truth of abundance once you fully understand all the various damaging, toxic, and limiting ways the 99% think.

Can you see how a deprivation mentality and a lack of confidence are linked? How they are both symptoms of the same underlying bad thinking?

HOW TO ACCESS YOUR ABUNDANCE

So now we've gone through all the ways that most people limit their abundance.

Next, I want to show you the simple things you can do to massively expand your abundance.

But before I explain this in a little more detail, I would like you to slow down and consider for a moment the key phrase I used earlier in this chapter and in this book.

Your default state is the state you're most often in.

The things I'm about to show you will shift your default state back to your natural childlike state where an abundant mindset was your default.

These things are the daily equivalent of cleaning your teeth. If you don't clean your teeth every day, they will quickly get yellowed, dirty, damaged, and breakdown.

Well, exactly the same is true of your mindset and the abundance that it brings you. You need to clean away the day-to-day build-up of bad thinking that damages your mindset and abundance thinking.

You are bombarded each day with the false and damaging thinking of the 99%. Without maintaining the simple and easy daily practices to keep your mind clean and in tune, you will fall back into the deprivation thinking that has blocked so much abundance from coming into your life already.

None of these things are hard work or require effort; they just gently shift your thinking, to tune in to and fully unleash your natural abundance.

RAISING YOUR CONSCIOUSNESS

First, you need to start tuning your mind to look for and see all the incredible abundance around you right now. The first step in this is simply raising your consciousness.

"Raising your consciousness" means raising *your awareness*, becoming aware (again) of the things that you have stopped being consciously aware of. In the context of abundance, that means seeing the higher truth of the abundance that was always there but that you had tuned out.

It means seeing the underlying truth of abundance despite the appearance of lack and deprivation.

It means looking for and seeing the endless abundance around you always.

Let me give you an example.

When a business mentor of mine was starting his (now extremely successful) business, he was almost out of money.

To the outside world, all appearances were of lack and deprivation. He had to sell his car, move into a tiny apartment, and his credit cards were pretty much maxed out.

He would seek out the most expensive hotels in London and sit in the lounges to work. He did this very consciously and deliberately. He knew that he was surrounded by abundance – he had raised his consciousness to that level. He deliberately put himself in places where he could see the incredible abundance around him.

He didn't just see the material abundance in wealthy, top-class hotels. He walked along the streets of London seeing the huge number of people (the abundance of people) he could be of service to – and who would reward him handsomely for his work.

He recognized that there was an overabundance of people who he could help. There was no lack. He only needed to tune his mind to access it.

He filled his mind with all the people across the world he could help, seeing how, at his fingertips, he had access to all those people, and how he only needed to connect and be of service to a tiny percentage of them in order to generate vast wealth for himself and those he loved.

Within a few weeks he had made his first sale; within a few months he was out of debt. Within 18 months he was a multimillionaire, staying in the hotels he had previously only been able to visit.

Can you see what he did here? He remained tuned into abundance. He saw the abundance in front of him despite the appearance of lack. He didn't allow all the negative, limiting thinking to block the conveyor belts of incredible supply and abundance to him.

He raised his consciousness to see abundance no matter what. _He remained clear that he was naturally an abundant being, as are you._

Each day, no matter your circumstances, take a few moments to see the abundance around you. It is there if you simply take a moment to look for it. Maybe if you're seeking material wealth, just observe the wealth around you; if you're seeking love and your perfect partner, look around and see all the love around you and for you. Know it is there.

See the abundance in nature. As I'm walking or driving along, I will just see how abundant nature is all around me. It reminds me that our natural state is of abundance.

YOU ARE AN ABUNDANT BEING

Remind yourself of the truth that you are an abundant being, that abundance is your birthright. I visualize the picture I described earlier of me being in that massive room as the center of a huge wonderful, magical factory warehouse. I watch all the conveyor belts go by.

I slow down and consider what blocks or limits I have unconsciously allowed in, that are restricting the abundance that is in front me.

I look at all the fears, limits, lack, or false sense of risk that I might feel. I observe it but don't ever judge myself for it. I am simply looking for any blocks I have put in my own way. If I find any, I still my mind and then look at them for value.

I then watch them fall away as I realize that they are false and inaccurate blocks and limitations.

I cannot tell you how many times after doing this that I have seen answers to problems emerge as if out of nowhere, opportunities only a few minutes earlier I couldn't see.

This is unleashing every level of abundance – life giving you everything you need on demand.

I also look for how I am blocking abundance by my sense of "should" when I have decided that what I desire can only come in a very specific form otherwise I'm discounting it.

So many times, I realize I have blocked off incredible things by being attached to a certain view of how they "should" be. And when I detach and open my mind to other possibilities, I so often receive something far bigger and better, way beyond my own view of what was "realistic."

Lastly, and very importantly, as a crucial part of me seeing myself as an abundant being, I realize that ***there is value and benefit in every situation I face.***

No matter how awful or bad it may ***appear,*** I know there is value and benefit. I know this is abundance appearing as lack. So, no matter what, I look for the value and benefit to me and ***it is always there.***

Most people miss the incredible life-changing value of so much that happens to them because they judge it by appearances instead of _seeing the truth in spite of appearances_.

But because I know that I am an abundant being, that everything that happens to me works out for the very best for me, I know that even the very worst situations are simply another form of abundance disguised as something that I don't want.

When you begin to see this underlying truth, everything that happens has value to you, propels you forward, takes you further towards creating the life that you want to live and becoming the person you want to be.

Just remember, you are an abundant being.

PRACTICING GRATITUDE

I've gone through the immense, transformative power of gratitude and the importance of having a daily gratitude practice.

This matters because without it your ego will hide away all the evidence of abundance, of the great, wonderful, and amazing things that happen to you all the time.

By keeping your gratitude list, by updating it each day with all the moments and things big and small that you are grateful for, you train your mind to stay tuned into abundance.

You are feeding your subconscious mind with data about the abundance you have in your life so that it retunes back to seeing abundance by default instead of deprivation and lack by default.

It is part of gently shifting your default state back to abundance.

Remember, your default state is the state you're most often in.

So, each of the practices puts you in the state of gratitude and tuned into abundance. This means you'll access more of the abundance available to you, and this gives you more reasons for gratitude and to be tuned into that abundance.

And so, a virtuous cycle of abundance is created on purpose instead of a deprivation cycle of lack being created by accident.

THINGS TO CONSIDER

- Do you expect abundance or lack and deprivation in your life? Don't answer straightaway. Consider this.

- Are you consciously or unconsciously allowing lack thoughts to dominate your thinking instead of remaining aware of the truth of abundance?

- Do you think you are deserving of abundance? If not, consider why not.

- Consider all the abundance around you right now, hiding in plain sight, whether in terms of material wealth, love, friendship, in nature, answers to problems. How much of this abundance had you become unconscious of?

- Consider that you can just as easily program your mind to tune into lack or abundance. Which would you prefer to be tuned into?

- Can you see how the ability to control your mind, to focus and direct your thoughts, is so critical to you remaining tuned into abundance instead of lack?

- Can you control your thoughts yet?

- How many of the different ways of creating lack – the shoulds, a belief in luck, through fears and self-imposed limits – have you unconsciously practiced in the past?

- Can you see the truth that you (like all of nature) are naturally abundant?

- Consider all the things that you have to be grateful for right now – friendships, love and connections, your partner, your children, opportunities you currently have, experiences you have had – and consider if lack or abundance is your underlying truth.

CHAPTER 18

THE POWER OF PERSPECTIVE

Nothing has any meaning in life except the meaning we give it.

TONY ROBBINS

I want to offer you a thought that most people dismiss completely.

And as a result, they deny themselves one of the most important secrets to changing their lives.

Observe your ego throw up all kinds of objections as you read what I'm about to tell you. And notice how your ego's need to be right might be getting in the way of you getting exactly what you want.

But if you consider and then accept the truth of this, your life will change dramatically.

Perception is more important than reality.

How you see yourself and the world around you, how you perceive yourself, events, people, situations, and circumstances determines what your life looks like way, way, way more than the underlying "truth" or "facts" of the events or people themselves.

Each and every experience we have is mediated through <u>our perception</u>: the lens, **the meaning**, we place upon those experiences.

What those events mean is therefore defined <u>within us</u>, not *out there*.

Two people can face exactly the same event, but their experience is often (in fact, usually) completely different. The difference is not "what happened," but each person's perception of it and the meaning they apply to it.

Let me give you an example.

Take an extreme sport like bungee jumping. Now this is not my thing *at all*, but plenty of people love it.

My perception and so my meaning of a bungee jump is that it's unpleasant, uncomfortable, and probably vomit inducing. You would need a small, highly trained army to get me to do one, let alone get me to actually pay for the experience.

For other people, it is quite literally the most exciting, wonderful, thrill-inducing thing they can think of. They pay good money to do it many times, and often the more extreme the experience the better.

The experience is exactly the same, but the perception (and so the meaning attached to it) is completely different.

Now think of the experience of failure.

Most people hate failing, **absolutely hate it**, and will do almost anything to avoid it.

I used to feel that way for many years. I was absolutely one of those "failure is not an option" people. (I am grateful that I have since learned how damaging this mindset is.)

If I tried something and it went "wrong," I would be angry, frustrated, upset, and usually give up. I would take it as a signal that something "wasn't for me."

My meaning was that failure was like getting a "D" on a test at school: that it was evidence that I was not good enough, defective, and didn't have the necessary talent.

Now I understand that experiencing failure is not only *an option* but *the only and best option* if I want to create the life I want to live and become the person I want to be.

I now actively look forward to *intelligently failing* at something, because I know that the treasure I will receive is vast. I will quite literally receive precisely the skills, experience, learning, and wisdom I need to progress to the next level in my life.

I now see experiencing failure as a wonderful, incredible gift.

Through a difference in perspective, the same event, sometimes for the same person leads, to an entirely different experience. Simply by seeing it differently.

HOW YOUR PERSPECTIVE LITERALLY CREATES YOUR REALITY

Can you see how your perspective <u>creates</u> your reality?

How, if you can control your perspective, you can, quite literally, control your reality.

And I mean control your reality in every meaningful, practical, real-life, get up in the morning and see the difference, sense.

The way to do this is to change the "truths" you know about yourself and the world around you.

Or, to put it more accurately and in a way that actually helps you, *change the stories that you've <u>decided are true</u> about yourself and the world around you.*

This whole book is really about how you see yourself and see the world.

Because mindset, confidence, and success are really just perception.

The first section of this book was all about revealing to you (by which I mean, making you conscious of) the false, toxic, damaging perspectives that most of us were taught as we grew up.

And, for 99% of people, that created a distorted, disfigured, inaccurate, and limited perspective of themselves, of the life available to them, and what the world really holds for them.

The second section of this book was about giving you back – _reconnecting you_ with – the natural confidence and success perspectives that you were born with but that got buried under layers and layers of limiting thinking and stifling social conditioning.

It was about peeling away the disempowering and unhelpful perspectives and replacing them with accurate, truthful, empowering ones.

When we begin to see ourselves and the world differently, we act differently. We make different choices; we walk through different doors; we connect with different people; and we feel completely different about who we are.

We naturally and without stress or strain do the same things as the 1% do. And as a result, we become the people we want to be and create the lives we want to live.

"I NEVER THOUGHT OF IT THAT WAY"

By changing the way we see ourselves and our situations and experiences, we transform not only what they mean but the impact they have on us.

You can change your perception of a situation, a problem or a challenge, or even a bad experience. It can be one that's happening now or one that's happened in your past.

And in doing so, it can go from being a limit to a liberator, from being something that holds you back to being something that propels you forward.

From being bulky baggage to priceless treasure.

This is how you become an alchemist in your own life *turning every experience into a valuable one.* Most people, though, do reverse alchemy, taking every experience and turning them into increasingly more hurt, pain, and baggage.

If you perceive every experience as a gift, no matter what appearances suggest, then that is what you will experience it as.

If you perceive experiences as pain and trauma, devoid of any good or benefit, that will just as easily become the "truth" of your experience.

Through so many of my conversations with my coach Stephen and with my friend and mentor Andy, there were countless "perception shift" moments, where previously bad experiences came to be seen as the gifts they were.

Where I came to see the truth about who I was and what I was capable of; where I saw clearly the false limits I had created for myself and the limiting labels I had given myself.

I saw for the first time that I had the power to change the meaning of any experience I had had; that I didn't have to be a prisoner to past perceptions and past labels; that I was free to choose new meanings and narratives that helped me instead of sticking with ones that harmed me.

Everything in this book has been designed to bring about that same perception shift in you, following the exact process and steps that I followed with these two great mentors.

And in doing so, the process is designed to set you free to unleash all the incredible potential, talents, and gifts that were always inside of you and available to you through every experience.

If you want to watch an incredibly powerful example of this, go onto YouTube and search for "Jo Ann Compton" on Oprah Winfrey.

Jo Ann Compton's 18-year-old daughter, Laurie Ann, was murdered. Like any parent, she suffered unimaginable pain and grief as a result of this truly horrific experience.

The show in question was around 10 years after her daughter's death. In that time, she had left her daughter's room untouched almost like a shrine. She had, in her own words, stopped living. It was like time simply wouldn't move forward. She was in so much pain that she wasn't able to be emotionally available for her other daughter.

It is very emotional to watch her speak to her pain and grief. She is clearly in incredible anguish.

She later opens up and admits that her intention was to go home after the show and take her own life.

Then something incredible happens that changes everything for her.

Dr. Phil, says to her, "If she [Laurie Ann] could talk to you right now, do you think she would say, 'Mother, I want you to hurt every day for the rest of your life to prove that you loved me?'"

It becomes clear that Jo Ann feels (i.e., her perception is) that it would be a betrayal of her daughter **not to remain in this grief** for the rest of her life. Her perception is that the depths of her love for her daughter is <u>evidenced by the depths of her pain.</u>

That if she lets go of the pain, she would somehow be saying that she no longer loved her daughter, that, somehow, she would no longer be honoring the memory of her daughter.

Then Dr. Phil says:

"Maybe the betrayal is focusing on the **day of her death** rather than **the event of her life**. She lived for 18 vibrant and wonderful years and yet you're focusing on the day that she died."

You can see in the video that Jo Ann is stunned. You can see the moment when, suddenly, everything has changed for her.

She says:

"I never thought of it that way. I really never thought of it that way."

Later in the video, there is a scene where she is interviewed again several years later by Oprah Winfrey and you can see a completely changed person. You see someone who is living again; someone who has reconnected with her other daughter; someone who has reconnected with <u>herself</u>; and someone whose life has changed beyond all recognition.

I share this with you because I want you to see the incredible reality-defining power of your perception; how, even in this most horrific, most awful of experiences, simply seeing the same situation with new eyes changes everything.

A shift in your perception can allow you to let go of incredible pain and embrace the awe-inspiring full potential of your life.

"HOW YOUR PERCEPTION CREATES WHO YOU BECOME"

First you make your beliefs, then your beliefs make you.

– MARISA PEER

That same reality-defining power applies just as much to how you <u>perceive external events</u> as it does to how you <u>perceive yourself</u>.

In the same way as we apply meanings to the things that happen, we apply meanings to ourselves – to who we perceive ourselves to be.

This creates our sense of "who we are."

And we act in accordance with those self-perceptions irrespective of whether they *<u>help us greatly or harm us terribly</u>*.

That sense of who we are defines precisely how far you will go in life – whether you will create the life of your dreams or a life that leaves you emptied out and uninspired.

With the right, true, and accurate sense of yourself, your potential and the potential for your life is essentially unlimited.

This is the way the 1% live and it is now the way that you, through reading, considering, and then most importantly *applying* the thought structures in this book are starting to live.

Only you can decide if you want to permanently join the 1% by making it a way of life.

As you've gone through the chapters of this book, you have, step-by-step been removing each layer of false, limited, and distorted perception about who you really are.

And with it you have shifted from a false disempowering sense of who you are to an accurate empowering one.

Most people's stories disempower and disable them. They stop them from even getting started. They ensure failure before they even begin making progress towards creating their dream life and towards becoming the person they desire to be.

That is because you always act in alignment with your perspective of who you are, no matter whether that perspective helps you or harms you.

The problem is that we aren't taught how to choose our perspective _consciously_.

And so, until we learn to control our thoughts (our perspective), our confidence and success in life is a matter of chance not choice.

YOUR TENDANCIES ARE NOT YOUR DESTINY

Have you mistaken who you are today, with who you are destined to be?

Have you decided, consciously or unconsciously, that who you will become and the life you will live is defined by who you perceive yourself to be today, right now, in this moment?

Or do you see, do you feel and know, the truth that the only person you are destined to become, the only life you are destined to live, is the one that you choose?

Everyone is born with natural, inherent tendencies – a tendency towards shyness and introversion, towards risk taking, towards being extrovert and social, towards fitting in or making the world adjust to who they are.

But these are only tendencies, and your tendencies are not your destiny.

This is a lie that most people get told and tell themselves. But it remains a lie nonetheless.

And one that keeps you trapped inside a set of false limitations that stop you living the life you want on your terms.

Changing them is simply a matter of realizing which tendencies help you and which ones hold you back from being who you want to be.

And then getting comfortable with being uncomfortable for a short period until the new way of being, the new tendency, stops feeling uncomfortable, then feels normal and then becomes your new default setting.

You have done this many times already, as you adapted to new challenges, new experiences, new environments. You have reprogrammed your default state many times over.

You have simply done it unconsciously, without realizing that you had.

Now imagine if you did that on purpose, in a directed way – in a way designed to help you become who you wanted to be and to create the life you want to live.

Imagine if you consciously chose to develop the tendencies, the default settings, that meant you inevitably created and lived your life exactly as you wished.

That is the choice you have now and have always had. And always will have. It is your choice to create your own destiny, consciously and on purpose.

THE LIE OF BEING BORN A "WINNER"

Next time you want to feel inspired, read about Nick Vujicic.

Nick was born with a rare disorder that has only six other recorded cases worldwide and meant he was born without limbs.

When he was first born his mother refused to hold him or even see him.

Despite the challenges of no limbs, of not being able to walk, of being bullied at school, Nick has achieved more than most people would even attempt let alone actually do.

He graduated from university with a double major.

He married and had four children.

He founded an international non-profit organization and ministry.

He launched his own motivational speaking company.

He starred in a short movie AND was awarded a best actor prize for his performance.

He created and launched a single and music video.

He has written numerous books.

He learned to swim and surf. <u>With no arms or legs</u>.

I don't want to tell you this so that you compare yourself to Nick in any way.

There is no value or benefit in comparing yourself to anyone. It only ever makes you feel bad and feeling bad never helps you to progress.

What I would like you to do, if you want to feel inspired and make progress, is see just how much you can achieve *if you don't accept the lies and false perceptions about who are you and what you can achieve*.

Just how much of a lie the perception of being born a winner or loser is. How much of a lie the perception of not being good enough is.

And just how much of a lie that sense that you are not worthy of success and all the good things in life is.

To see the incredible power you have; to <u>create</u> the quality of your life.

No matter what, <u>literally no matter what</u>, you can achieve truly staggering, incredible things.

Your dreams are entirely within your reach. You can. Full stop. End of story.

HOW YOUR PERCEPTION CREATES YOUR LIFE

Life is a reflection of what you think. If your thoughts are negative, the world you see will be the same.

– LEON BROWN

Your life is a reflection of your thinking.

Despite most people knowing this truth, 99% of the world spends most of their time thinking predominantly negative thoughts.

You cannot create the life you want or become the person you want to be with a mind filled with negativity.

Negative thoughts create negative emotions, which in turn produce negative actions.

Those negative actions will only create more things to feel negative about. And so a downward spiral is created.

Focus on things that are shit and you will get more shit things to focus on.

Focus on the incredible, exciting possibilities for your life, leaving no space in your mind for negativity, and your life will fill up with excitement and possibility.

Become conscious of the negative thoughts you allow into your mind – the irritation, anger, impatience, resentment, envy, etc. – and ask yourself if they are helping you in any way.

When you realize the truth that every negative thought in some way holds you back, they will become very easy to drop.

Let me give you an example, a big one: happiness. Your perspective of yourself and the world directly determines your sense of how happy you are. It has very, very little to do with the facts of your life, despite what most people think.

The problem is that most people misunderstand happiness.

Most people think you can only be happy when you get "there"; when you've got the relationship, got the money, got the house, booked the holiday, etc.

But that's pleasure NOT happiness.

Don't misunderstand me, there's nothing wrong with pleasure **at all**. I love pleasure and I love the "stuff." But it isn't the same as happiness.

And because of that misunderstanding, the bad teaching and backwards thinking that says happiness arrives when you get "there," most people are trapped in misery.

But "there" isn't a place. It's a feeling.

You get that feeling not from external "stuff" but from your focus, from your perception of yourself and your life.

By focusing on all the amazing things that you have in your life, instead of on the things that you think are wrong or missing.

If you're not happy now, I absolutely 100% guarantee you won't be when you get the stuff.

Happiness comes from recognizing the truth that you are complete right now and the stuff will simply add more pleasure to your life.

Your ego will be likely telling you that I am full of shit right now.

But ask yourself how many truly happy people you know and examine how many of them are really the people with all the stuff, instead of simply the right focus.

And don't let your ego tell you that by allowing yourself to be happy now, that somehow that will make you lazy or slack about achieving your dreams. That is bullshit that your ego uses to stop you from EVER being happy.

Dissatisfaction and unhappiness are not (despite what so many think) prerequisites for success.

Happiness with who you are and your life right now, no matter what, is an essential part of confidence.

So stop putting off your happiness. Enjoy your life right now.

HOW TO CHANGE YOUR PERCEPTION SO THAT IT HELPS YOU INSTEAD OF HARMING YOU

Thinking is the hardest work there is, which is probably the reason so few engage in it.

– HENRY FORD

Your perspective is created by your focus.

What you focus on creates your dominant thoughts and it is your dominant thoughts that create your perspective.

The more you focus on thinking the thoughts that help you instead of the thoughts that harm you, the more your confidence and success will grow. And equally and just as easily, the more you focus on thoughts that harm you, the more your lack of success and confidence will grow.

That's why I have emphasized over and over in this book the foundational importance of learning to control your thoughts.

So just before we continue, slow down and ask yourself if you have yet learned this foundational skill, the skill without which you cannot create sustainable lasting success.

Don't feel bad if you haven't. But do recognize that the value of everything else you have learned here will be lost if you don't make it your key priority to learn this master skill – the skill that as Tim Ferriss says is the "meta-skill," the skill that unlocks all others.

Because it is only when you master control of your thoughts that you can, on demand, choose your focus and so master your perspective.

So, stop and consider now, right now in this moment: Where's your focus?

Do you focus on the one and only thing you have complete control over, the thoughts in your mind? And so becoming the very best version of you?

Or do you focus on what's "wrong" **with the world around you** and make yourself a victim of circumstance?

There's a very, very big difference between those who live a life of happiness, success, confidence, and abundance and those who do not.

The people who succeed are those who focus on who they need to be in order to live the life they want.

They're focused on the circumstances inside of themselves and they spend time each day becoming the best version of themselves: calm, happy, confident, grateful, unshakeable.

And as a result they like, respect, and love who they are. They enjoy being the person they are.

And so, no matter the external circumstances they face, life is good.

But just as importantly, because their dominant focus and state is content, happy, and grateful this is the lens through which they see the outside world.

So they see wonderful possibilities where others only see closed doors.

They see abundance where others see lack. And they are able to create a life that makes sense to them no matter the circumstances they face.

Ninety-nine percent of people focus on the external world.

They blame external events, people, and situations for the state of their lives.

They seek out new opportunities to blame, to hand over responsibility for their lives, to find excuses.

But they miss the critical point which is that none of that blame, none of those excuses, takes you a single step closer to your dreams.

In the end the only work that any of us really have to do is to become a better version of ourselves.

So where will your focus be today?

THINGS TO CONSIDER

- Can you see how your perception defines your reality? Have you considered the power that this gives you?

- Can you see how two people can experience precisely the same situation or circumstances and perceive it differently? Some will perceive it in ways that weaken them and others in ways that empower and strengthen them. How will you now choose to perceive the next challenge you face?

- Consider how seeing events from your past in new ways completely changes the meaning of those events – and how you see yourself as a result. Which events from your past will you now choose to see differently?

- Consider that having the ability to choose your perception makes you an alchemist. It gives you the ability to turn every experience into something of value.

- Have you made yourself a prisoner of past labels and perceptions that don't serve you? Consider: Would you like to change any of these now?

- Can you see the good in yourself as clearly as the faults?

- Consider that your perception of yourself and your world is created by your dominant thoughts. Will you decide to master control of your thinking so that you can create the perceptions that help you?

FREE GIFT # 3 – BONUS LESSON: "CREATING THE PLAN FOR YOUR LIFE"

If you want to go deeper on creating your life by design
and see the exact steps I use with my private clients to
create the life they were always meant to be living – go to
www.unstoppableselfconfidence.com/confidence-on-demand
and watch "Creating The Plan For Your Life" where I run through
this blueprint step-by-step. I've also included a free worksheet to
help you create the plan for your life on your terms. It's absolutely
free. Enjoy.

LIVING LIFE ON YOUR TERMS

CHAPTER 19

THE STEPS TO BECOME UNSTOPPABLE

> **You have greatness within you, and responsibility to manifest that greatness.**
>
> LES BROWN

This is the final chapter on installing the right thinking.

We'll be going through the last few thought structures that you need to live life on your terms. These are the ways of thinking that help you as you actually step forward onto your journey to the life that you want.

I designed this book to create real and lasting change in the people who read it. I didn't want people to read it and think, "That was great, I feel amazing" and then do nothing with the knowledge.

That's a waste of your time and mine.

You only unlock the value of the knowledge this book contains when you apply it, when you use it as your guide on your journey.

This chapter deals with the tools you need as you get started: how you deal with the obstacles and challenges you meet along your journey so that you stay on track until your dream life has become your reality.

WHY YOU HAVE A RESPONSIBILITY
TO BECOME THE BEST YOU

But first let me tell you a short story to explain why unleashing your greatness and achieving the success and confidence you desire matters so much to me.

When I was working with Stephen, we talked a lot about what makes relationships thrive and what causes them to fail.

He told me something that profoundly impacted me and that was the inspiration for my journey with *Unstoppable Self-Confidence*.

It is the reason that you are reading this book now – because I recognized that what he was telling me was one of those incredibly simple but profound truths that **changes everything**.

Let me explain.

Stephen said that when nearly all couples come to see him, he is almost certainly dealing with pretty much the worst version of each person in the relationship.

At the start of the relationship, when they fell in love and when things felt amazing, they were being great versions of themselves. And so, the relationship makes each person feel wonderful within it.

Over time, as they encounter changes, challenges, and problems (and they don't have the framework or tools to deal with them in ways that strengthen the relationship instead of weakening it), each person tends to become a lesser version of themselves in the relationship.

This changes the dynamic within the relationship, so that each person withdraws a little and becomes a little more disconnected because they no longer feel wonderful. They feel a little less safe and a little less loved.

Eventually, unless they find ways to deal with these challenges, the relationship falls into decline and crisis. One or both people end up operating in that relationship as the worst versions of themselves: scared, fearful, angry, hurt, and causing each other pain.

Is it any surprise then, he asked me, that these relationships are in deep trouble?

Is it a surprise that these relationships are a cause of pain instead of happiness, beset by arguments, resentments, toxic behaviors, affairs, and many other things besides?

But the truth about the relationship isn't defined by the state of the relationship when both people are existing as the worst versions of themselves. Any relationship would be challenged in those circumstances.

The truth about the relationship (and the people within it) comes from when they operate _as the best versions of themselves_ with the tools and frameworks to deal with the challenges they face.

When they unleash their greatness within the relationship. No matter what.

When they remain true to the very best of themselves even when the other person is struggling or behaving poorly.

They do this because they realize that this is who they really are.

Stephen told me that initially both parties want to express the pain they feel, the hurt within them that they feel has been caused by their partner. They want to explain the situations that have caused them pain.

But can you see how pointless it would be to try to improve these relationships by simply dealing with the "presenting symptoms"?

Unless and until you change the version of the people operating in the relationship from awful to good and then to great, the same or slightly different symptoms will continue.

Until each individual changes their focus to being their best self no matter what, they will simply **take the same challenges into the next relationship**.

The great relationship that both people really want – passionate, connected, sexual, with respect, love, and the freedom to be all of who they are – only comes when both people operate as the best of themselves in the relationship.

This is where the reality of Einstein's wonderful quote that "no problem can be solved from the same level of consciousness that created it" matters.

By raising the consciousness of both people in the relationship, the problems get solved.

Now when I explain this example to most people, they get it and understand how it solves that problem.

But here's what most people miss.

Through that process of change, they don't just become better partners. They become better people: better parents, better friends, better brothers, sisters, uncles, aunts, work colleagues, better to themselves. Because they are operating at a higher level of their true potential.

And the ripples of positive change that flow from them unleashing their greatness impact all of their interactions, all of the situations they are involved in, all of the people they engage with.

The more people unleash their greatness, the more problems simply fall away. Because more and more people are operating at a different level of consciousness.

Now I want you to picture in your mind all 7 billion people who live on the planet today. Imagine each of them with a monitor above their heads showing the level of their true potential they have reached.

How many people do you feel are operating anywhere near their true potential? How many of the challenges you see around you would simply fall away if most people operated at their best instead of at their worst?

Can you see how it is not just within your reach to live your best life **but also your responsibility?**

That you living your best life as the best version of you inspires others to start doing the same.

And as a direct result, more and more of the problems you see around simply dissolve. They fall away because the conditions they need to survive no longer exist.

This is the equivalent of becoming healthy. By eating right, by exercising right, by eliminating the bad foods and drink, your health improves all around. The conditions of your body are no longer supportive for illness, only for health.

So, you are no longer trying to cure disease; you have instead <u>created wellness</u>.

In exactly the same way, being the best you creates a vibrant, healthy life so that you <u>not only solve the problems you think you face, but you create the conditions where those problems can no longer exist</u>.

And you show others the benefits of doing the same through every interaction with you.

This was the message that Stephen gave me. And it is the message I want to share with you.

You have greatness within you. And everyone benefits when you unleash it.

THE MAGIC INGREDIENT FOR SUCCESS

In an earlier chapter I talked through how numerous studies have shown that the shorter the time between learning something and applying it, the greater your chances are of achieving success.

In exactly the same way: the shorter the time between making a decision and acting upon that decision, the greater your chances of success.

That is because momentum is the key to success.

The shorter the gap, the more likely you are to first actually take action and second to get the immediate feedback on that action that inspires you to do more.

That is, you are more likely to create momentum instead of dissipating it.

Each moment wasted is a moment where you can start to overthink what might happen instead of finding out what actually does happen. Where your ego can start to fill your mind with doubts instead of possibilities. Where you lose the opportunity to gain real-life learning (the only learning that really matters), to gain the true skills, wisdom, and experience you need to achieve your goals **instead of just the theory of them**.

This is because the very fastest way to learn what you need to learn, to get the wisdom, skills, and experience you need to create the life you want comes from applying and living the knowledge you have learned, not just intellectually processing it.

This is *real-life learning* as opposed to *academic learning*. And it is the natural model of success.

Most people when they decide to say start a business, will go and do research, go and do a course, go and read a book, go and talk to lots of people, go and do almost anything other than actually starting the business itself, other than making their first sale.

Andy Shaw is the most remarkably talented person I know for getting businesses started and he has done it in multiple different fields, making millions along the way.

He told me that the model for success he uses is *Ready, Fire, Aim.*

What he means by this is that he will often make sales for a new business before he has really got started. He makes the sales to know that he will get paid for his efforts and that the demand exists for whatever he is selling.

But by making the sales up front, he has created momentum behind the business. He can see the value that he will be creating for his customers, for his partners, and for himself.

Now, he may (and usually does) spend a reasonable amount of time considering what businesses he wants to do, how they will work, what he will offer and so on.

But once he reaches the decision to go ahead, he takes action fast. **Very fast**. He has thought slowly so that he can act really quickly.

He identifies the first step to do and gets on with it straightaway. Only once that step is complete will he take the next step and then the next and then the next.

He works diligently in a workmanlike way on the task he has to do next and only that task until it is done. Each task completed is another building block of momentum.

While he does research and due diligence before he gets started, he knows that once *the decision to proceed has been made*, it is critical to build momentum.

Most people take their energy and divert it into almost anything other than building the business *and so dissipate their momentum instead of building it*. And waste a huge amount of time, money, and energy in the process.

I learned this lesson very painfully and it is one I am always very, very conscious never to repeat.

Several years ago, I was starting a business and needed to raise about $500K in investor finance. I was so "enthusiastic" about getting started I immediately booked a course about how to raise money. I then bought a bunch of books on how to raise finance and how to pitch my idea to investors. I watched episodes of Dragons' Den (or Shark Tank in the US). And eventually, after a few months, I went out and tried to get my first round of money.

And guess what happened? <u>Nothing, zero, zilch. I bombed</u>.

Looking back, I can see how important that experience was for me. Because I had <u>wasted so much time getting to the point of simply getting started that I hadn't experienced the reality of raising money, only the theory of it</u>.

Only once I got started did the real learning begin.

Only by going through meetings where I kept getting turned down could I learn what investors really wanted as opposed to what the books and courses said that they wanted.

Through each failure, I learned a little more, refined my pitch, got better prepared with answers to questions that I had never previously considered. I was learning each time, getting better, more experienced, and more skillful.

It took me about 25 meetings to raise my first round of money and only a relatively small slice at about $20K. It took another five meetings to raise the remaining $480K.

The reason was that I had created momentum.

Even the people who turned me down were often willing to introduce me to other investors who might be interested – and so my network of contacts expanded. I went from being nervous and unsure of how to answer some questions to being completely sure of how to answer any question.

All of that came from getting out there and doing real-life learning, and so creating momentum instead of destroying it.

BEING WILLING TO BEING A BEGINNER

One of the biggest myths (lies) that stops most people going after their dreams is that they are not yet an "expert."

That they don't "know enough;" that they don't have enough experience; that they haven't yet acquired the skills they need in order to succeed.

And so they decide not to even get started.

Which is of course the one and only **absolutely guaranteed** way to ensure that you will never become an expert.

Yet, this way of thinking overlooks the clear and obvious fact the no one is born an expert in anything.

That the only way to become an expert is to start: to start learning, to start applying, to start practicing, making mistakes, and refining your craft. That is how the process of mastery (becoming an expert) works.

Our egos like to trap us by telling us that we must become an expert before we start. But then when you become an expert in one area, our egos simply shift the goalposts and tell us that we're not an expert in some other area.

And the cycle continues until we become exhausted, worn out, and give up. And so, our egos have ensured that no progress was made and another person's dreams have died.

The true measure is not whether you are an expert, but whether you know the (very small) amount needed **to just get started**.

Today, if you want to, set yourself free of the idea that you need to be an expert to get started.

Instead, realize the truth that your success is based on your level of momentum, not on your level of expertise.

MAINTAINING MOMENTUM

The size of your success is measured by the strength of your desire, the size of your dream, and how you handle disappointment along the way,

– ROBERT KIYOSAKI

One of the misconceptions about success is that it happens in a straight line.

That you simply decide where you want to get to, set off, and find your way there.

The reality is very different, as almost anyone who has achieved massive success will tell you.

They will, almost without exception, talk to the challenges and obstacles they faced along the way. They will speak of the periods of struggle and frustration followed by sudden leaps forward.

They will say how, very often, they fell backwards before they took their biggest steps forward.

The difference between those who make it and those who do not, is that the successful 1% know that what the world calls struggle is simply part of the journey.

That the path to success isn't a straight line at all.

But rather an adventure-filled, meandering, twisty path with obstacles along the way. Each obstacle is a gateway, where you face a choice to give up and turn back or to learn what's needed to carry on. At the first sign of struggle, 99% of people turn back.

They see the struggle as a sign that this isn't the path for them as it isn't easy and straightforward.

The 1% see the truth that each struggle is a precious gift containing incredible value for you; that each struggle contains the lessons and experiences you need to progress to the next stage of your journey to the life you desire.

Your struggles don't make you a failure. In fact, nothing could be further from the truth.

They mean you are on the journey to inevitable success.

REMEMBER: PROBLEMS ARE JUST
SITUATIONS TO BE DEALT WITH

So how do you think this way consistently even when you hit challenges or problems?

Your ego will catch you off guard at some point and will try to seduce you with the old ways of thinking that keep you stuck, so there are a few really powerful thought structures I want to give you here to deal with these situations.

Your ego will try to tell you, in binary terms, that you haven't gotten this mindset at all; that you've gone backwards.

So first, I want you to remember to detach and observe these thoughts, to remain conscious to scan for them.

Remember, all change comes from being the non-judgmental observer of self. Don't let your ego skip you past the **non-judgmental observer** part there. Slow down and consider that for a few moments.

When something happens, when you feel thrown off-balance, slow down and realize that you haven't gone backwards at all; that, in fact, you are simply being offered new challenges and new ways to grow, expand, and reinforce your powerful new mindset.

Be delighted that you've noticed you're feeling off-balance because from that point you can make the changes you need to.

Then go back, as always, to the core foundational skill: to get back in control of your mind. To give yourself 15 seconds of positive thought and some moments of No Mind so that you are back in control of your thinking.

Then realize the truth that whatever you're facing is "**just a situation to deal with**."

Not a catastrophe; not a disaster; not some abyss that you will never escape from. Just a situation to deal with.

I have used this thought structure on countless occasions on my journey to creating my dream life. I have used it to deal with financial challenges, bureaucratic problems that seemed insurmountable, and at times when I have felt like my progress was blocked and I wasn't making progress "fast enough."

I stilled my mind, got back in control of my thinking, and recognized that this was just a situation to deal with.

And then I was free to calmly and in a workmanlike way, work through the problem I was dealing with.

Each time I did, I took a moment to realize that I had just grown a little stronger, a little more prepared for the journey ahead, and I felt delighted with myself.

And that by dealing with it, no matter what happened, I would be stronger, wiser, more experienced, and better equipped.

The second thought structure is to **expect problems to resolve themselves**.

Notice that I didn't say "hope problems would resolve themselves"; I said expect.

This is incredibly powerful and here's why: when you shift your thinking to expecting problems to solve themselves, you put your mind into a different level of thinking.

Your thinking shifts from doubt to certainty; you know with 100% certainty that the problem will get solved. It's simply a question of exactly how and exactly when.

As always, the real shift comes from when you realize that you do this already in the areas of your life where you are already naturally successful.

So, imagine for a second that you're stuck somewhere in a traffic jam, a bad traffic jam. You might be irritated, pissed off, or even a little angry. But do you really have any doubt at all that you will ultimately deal with the situation in front of you?

Sure, it may take longer than you planned to get where you're going, but you expect to get there. Rather than stressing about whether or not you will make it, because you expect the situation to get resolved one way or another, your mind quickly starts thinking of alternative solutions: different routes, whether to stop for a coffee and let the traffic pass, some people you need to call.

And soon enough, you find your way to your destination.

Well, this is no different from the challenges you face along your journey through life.

But here's what I've found to be even more powerful. When I've stilled my mind and expected the problem to get resolved, often all I need to do is stop and do nothing. And more often than you may imagine, the problem has simply fallen away.

Someone has come to me with a solution, the answer has just appeared, the circumstances that caused the problem in the first place have changed. And so, the problem no longer exists.

This is the power of expectation instead of hope.

The size of your problems is nothing compared to your ability to solve them.

Sometimes it's easy to feel overwhelmed by the problems we think we face: financial problems, job problems, relationship problems, health problems. And sometimes all of them at once.

But never underestimate your ability to not only solve these problems but actually thrive off the back of them.

You have hidden talents, strengths, resilience, and genius. *Adversity reveals these talents; comfortable ease hides them away and they atrophy.*

If you truly understood the breathtaking scope of what you are capable of, you wouldn't fear any problem. You would know the truth that you can handle this and any other challenge life throws at you.

The trick is to calm your mind and avoid judging what the problem "means" for you, your life, and for those you care about.

Instead, simply see possible ways the problem could (not definitely will, simply could) be solved.

And then in a calm, resolute, workmanlike way, just get on and do what is necessary to make your chosen outcome the reality.

But always be open to the possibility that what you see as a problem is actually life leading you somewhere better, even if it doesn't appear that way at the time.

Read the stories of the adversity that so many have faced.

And see the truth that their eventual far greater success come about precisely because of the challenges they faced.

EXCELLENCE AS A WAY OF LIFE

I'm an overnight success after 10 ten years.

– RAY KROC

The way to build evermore momentum towards your dream life is to focus on simply taking one step forward every day.

To become a little bit better than you were the day before.

What have you done today to make your life a little better than it was yesterday?

To move a little closer to becoming the person you want to be?

To improve your mindset, your health, your wealth, your relationships? To bring your goals and desires a little more into reality?

This question matters because one of the biggest myths that most of the world believes is that success is achieved in one big leap. When, in fact, success in anything comes through taking lots of small steps, building your life piece by piece every single day.

Then, eventually, to the outside world, it appears as if you've become successful overnight – when in fact that accumulation of all those steps simply made you reach the tipping point where your success became inevitable.

Sometimes that takes days, sometimes weeks, sometimes months, and sometimes years.

But the process is the same.

That's why if you're not moving forward, you're going against the natural process of success. You're sabotaging your ultimate success, you may simply be doing it unconsciously.

Success adds up; it builds up over time.

You learn one skill, and then master it. Then another. You get one thing done, and then another.

Over time, this builds an incredible platform of skills and experience that make your success inevitable.

But it only happens when each day you focus on moving forward, even if just a little bit.

So consider today, if you want to, what are you doing today to take that small step forward.

And so make your dreams inevitable.

THINGS TO CONSIDER

- Consider the truth that you have greatness within you waiting to be unleashed, and that the very best thing you can do for yourself, for those you love, and the wider world is to unleash it.

- Can you see the transformative power of becoming and living as the very best version of you? Consider what this means for your life.

- Take a few moments to consider the power of Einstein's wonderful quote, that "no problem can be solved from the same level of consciousness that created it. Instead of "trying" to solve problems, you could instead work on your mindset so that the problems could no longer exist.

- Consider the power of real-life learning instead of theoretical learning. Consider which type of learning gets you to the life you desire most effectively.

- Can you see that momentum is the magic ingredient for success?

- Consider the possibilities for your life that result from you once again being willing to be a beginner – just like when you were a young child and achieved the most incredible things.

- Can you see that the challenges and obstacles you face are gateways to you getting to the next level in your life and in your growth?

- Consider that problems are just situations to deal with.

CHAPTER 20

SO, WHAT WILL YOU DO NOW?

> Remembering that I'll be dead soon is the most important tool I've ever encountered to help me make the big choices in life. Because almost everything – all external expectations, all pride, all fear of embarrassment or failure – these things just fall away in the face of death, leaving only what is truly important. Remembering that you are going to die is the best way I know to avoid the trap of thinking you have something to lose. You are already naked. There is no reason not to follow your heart.
>
> STEVE JOBS

The purpose of this book is to reveal to you the truth about who you are and the power you hold in your hands to create your life by design.

To dispel the lies and myths that keep so many people trapped in lives of quiet desperation and the misery of false limitations – limitations that so many only understand to be lies when it's too late.

The waste of life is shocking.

But you now have a different choice and a completely different path open to you. Because you now understand that the truth is that you are not broken and you never were. Hardwired into your DNA is the truth that you are naturally confident and successful with everything you need to become exactly who you want to be and to create the life you want to live.

You now know that *confidence and success are a process, a choice*, and you now have everything you need to make that choice and, more importantly, to live that choice.

You have found truths about yourself, truths that place in your hands the power to create your life and the feelings of natural confidence <u>on demand</u>.

I want to show you the person you have now become, through reading, considering, and then applying the material and techniques contained in this book. I want you to fully grasp the incredible power you now have. Because now, even now, I want you to be conscious of how your ego will try to hide these powers from you.

In the first section, you came to see the most powerful, liberating truth of all: that there's nothing wrong with you; that you're not broken; and that you don't need fixing; <u>that any lack of confidence or success flowed not from who you are but what you were taught</u> – it flowed from lies and illusions that were designed to keep you stuck and playing small.

You felt the weight and baggage that had held you back for years fall away when you saw this simple but powerful truth.

The truth that who you are (always were and always will be) is astonishing beyond measure.

And so, you realized that you didn't need to **change away** from who you "really are" to become confident and successful. You only needed to **change back to the real you**. And in that identity flip, all the limiting lies and bullshit social conditioning that blocked and sabotaged your success began to fall away.

You reconnected with the real you, instead of thinking that the real you was your ego. And you saw that the things you didn't like about yourself were in fact the things you didn't like you about your ego – the negative voice in your head made up of all the bad programming, fears, and limits that those around "gifted" to you.

You learned the foundational skill for success in anything, the skill Tim Ferriss calls the "meta-skill" in that it unlocks all others: <u>the power to control your mind and so to think (and only think) thoughts that help you instead of thoughts that harm you</u>.

You are now able to control your mind on demand. When others lose control, you know exactly what to do so that you can unleash the incredible power of your subconscious mind to solve any problem. You have the ability to be in the world but separate from it at the same time, completely unfazed by the insanity you see around you.

In section two, you saw the real possibilities for your life, the real power you always held in your hands but was hidden from you by your ego and the bad teaching you were programmed with as you grew up.

You removed all the obstacles to unleashing your natural confidence and success mindset: fear, doubt, worry, approval seeking, perfectionism. You now see these as a pointless, destructive waste of time and so they have no place in your life.

You now understand that the process of failure is the master key to getting what you want. Where others dread and fear this, you now understand the natural model of learning, success, and then mastery is to do, fail, observe, and consider the lessons, and then redo, *applying the lessons*. Rinse and repeat.

You know how most of the world only ever looks at one side of a risk and so gets stuck because of the "safe problem," where they think they are playing it safe without seeing the incredible risks they are taking with their precious lives.

You know the incredible difference between **knowing** something and

believing it, and you know that belief and hope are nonsense – ideas that are no less insane despite the fact that 99% of people use them every day.

In section three, once you were free of the bad programming, you relearned your natural success and confidence mindset. And as a result, you've become a completely different person.

You've become the real you, the person you always really were: talented, gifted, powerful, capable, naturally fearless, and carefree; at peace with yourself and the world because your security comes from **who you are not what you have**. And so, you know you'll be just fine, no matter what.

Your focus, your mindset, has shifted from _consequence to possibility_ because you know that life always works out for the best for you even if it sometimes comes disguised as something you don't want or didn't plan for. But because you know that and because you are now the master of your mind instead of its slave, you simply look for all the ways any and every situation could (not definitely will) work out for the best for you.

You figured out for the first time in years who you really were and what you really wanted your life to be like – not what it should be like, but what you authentically desired it to be.

You are **inspired** by the vision you have in your mind for your life and you have learned how to design your life and everything you want in it so that you know with 100% certainty that it is how your future will turn out.

While others can't understand how you can be so certain, you know it has simply already happened and all you are doing is creating that certain picture in everyone else's reality.

You found your life purpose and that, along with you knowing your values and knowing what you want, means that decision-making is easy. Because every decision takes you towards your desires and aligns with your values or doesn't.

And lastly, where the world sees lack and deprivation, because you can control your mind and see the truth, you know that abundance is everywhere; that it is something you tune into. You see the truth about abundance that it isn't only material wealth, but the answer to every problem, the addressing of every need, the situations and circumstances that lead to your highest good, no matter appearances.

So, you can see the truth of abundance even when others see only lack.

A WORD OF WARNING

You have to build systems to protect against your lesser self.

– NEIL STRAUSS

I want to emphasize something really important. **And I do mean really important**.

You know all of this incredible wisdom now, but "knowing" is only ever a temporary state, as my brilliant friend Andy Shaw taught me. You can unlearn this all over again.

The bad programming is still out there and the wider world will try to drag you back into the insanity whenever it can.

One of the most important reasons that I wrote this book, post daily content online, and make my work so central to my day-to-day life is to protect myself against <u>unlearning</u> this incredible, precious knowledge.

I have created systems to protect against my lesser self because living as my lesser self has cost me so much.

So, no matter what, and I mean no matter what, every morning I spend 15–20 minutes bringing in the 15 seconds of positive thought, adding to or reviewing my gratitude list, and bringing in No Mind, ensuring that I start my day with a calm, grateful, happy mindset.

I have reminders set on my phone to bring in No Mind every couple of hours.

I read, listen to, or watch Andy Shaw's books, videos, or audio whenever I travel. Now I want to be clear that I have listened to his books at least 50 times all the way through. But I still learn things, gain new understanding, and remain in tune through this daily practice.

I read through my notes from my sessions with Stephen constantly. I have literally lost count of the number of times I have read them. But each time, I find something new, a deeper level of understanding. Any time I feel the need to retune my mind I delve straight back into these two sources.

I have had a few occasions where my ego has drawn me away from this way of life only for a day or so at most and it astonishes me how quickly the ways of the 99% can start to inflict all kinds of lack and damage.

And how quickly peace, abundance, and serenity return when I recognize this and go straight back to using the 15 seconds of positive thought, No Mind, and gratitude.

As Thomas Jefferson so wisely said, "The price of freedom is eternal vigilance."

However, I would prefer to reword this so that it gives you exactly what you need to stay on this path.

Instead, I would say that the price of freedom is eternal <u>consciousness</u>.

You have to remain conscious of when you start to feel bad or when the incredible feelings that you have gained through this book are not there in the same way. Once you have experienced it, it is easy to recognize when it's missing.

And you now know the path back. When it happens, remember there is no value in you feeling bad.

Your ego will instantly try to sabotage your journey by telling you that "you've gone backwards"; that "you're a fraud" for thinking that you'd got this; that "you're not really naturally confident and successful."

It will try to get you to focus on the short amount of time you slightly drifted off course instead of on the incredible benefits you have gained by being on course more of the time.

THIS ISN'T A BOOK TO BE READ ONCE

As I said at the start of this book, this isn't a book you only read once. This book is here for you to read and reread **_until_** you live this as a way of life, and then to refer back to as you need to, to maintain that way of life.

I've mentioned that I've read Andy Shaw's books (or listened to the audio versions) more than 50 times. It will be double that in the next year or so. Andy's book and my notes from my session with Stephen are things that I refer to over and over again.

This is no different to brushing your teeth. You can't just do it once. **_It is a way of life_**. Because this is about maintaining the right ways of thinking and living. But each time you do, your mind isn't simply staying at the same level – it is getting stronger and stronger.

This means that your ability to create grows more and more powerful, until you are "one of those people" who everyone looks at and just says, "_Well it's alright for them, everything just works out for them_."

EMBRACING YOUR NEW LIFE

The only thing you know with 100% certainty is that you have this life.

And that this life is a gift, a precious and rare gift.

Each day in your life is a gift, a chance to define who you really are and live a life that you're proud of. Ninety-nine percent of people squander this gift. Completely.

They casually and unconsciously waste their time instead of investing it.

They waste their lives through the fear of what others might think of them and their choices.

They play safe and small, not realizing (really realizing) that one day there will be no more "one days."

That one day they will no longer have the chance to live the life they dream of. That opportunity will be gone.

That one day they will no longer have the chance to live fully, authentically, and without apology as they are. To become the very best version of themselves.

That chance too will one day be gone.

I don't say any of this to make you feel bad. There is no benefit in that and I am only ever interested in that which benefits you.

I say it to make you conscious of choices most people only ever make **UNCONSCIOUSLY**. That is to say by accident instead of on purpose.

To give you the chance to grasp the wonderful gift you have in your hands right now.

To live fully, completely, joyfully, authentically – to live confidently.

That is a choice you make right now, whether you see it or not.

Each day you make the bold choice is a triumph. A triumph not just for you but for those around you.

Each day you play safe and small is a tragedy. A day you withhold from the world your incredible gifts and potential.

Today, go all in on your life. Go all in on you.

Your life is too precious to do anything else.

BONUSES TO SUPERCHARGE YOUR CONFIDENCE & SUCCESS

RECOMMENDED READING
& LINKS

I am often asked if there are other books or websites I would recommend to help people. I am usually very careful about this because it is all too easy to focus on simply reading more books and doing more courses.

And no matter how good those books or courses are, the greatest value you will ever get is by applying them and then living them as a way of life.

Applying what you have already read is 1,000 times more powerful and more valuable to you than reading another book.

Watch your ego trying to speed you away from what you have just read (and are almost certainly not yet living as a way of life) in order to find the next book.

- **Andy Shaw,** *Creating a Bug Free Mind* **and** *Using a Bug Free Mind* – I have often said that I struggle to fully articulate what Andy has done for me and the incredible impact he has had on my life. Andy taught me the framework for a successful life and his teachings are the inspiration for much of the material in this book. He showed me how to apply that framework to my life during one of the most difficult times I could have imagined. I have read and listened to these books more than 50 times. I cannot recommend them highly enough.

- **Stephen Hedger (www.stephenhedger.com)** – Stephen showed me the path back to myself, *to my best self*, and unleashed within me talents and greatness that I didn't know existed. Stephen showed me who I really was, that I wasn't broken and didn't need fixing. He showed me the truth that changed the path of my life: that I didn't need to learn to become confident and successful, that I simply needed to unlearn all the toxic, damaging nonsense that was blocking my natural confidence and success mindset. He showed me that the path to my dream life was through becoming and living as the very best version of myself in every situation no matter what.

- **Carol Dweck, *Mindset*** – This is a brilliant book for helping you realize the truth about just how powerful you are, and that success is a process, not a special gift for the select few.

- **Dr. Robert Glover, *No More Mr. Nice Guy*** – Don't be fooled by the title. This book is just as relevant for women as for men. I planned to just read the first few pages of this book to see what it was like. I didn't stop reading until I'd read it cover to cover. This book brilliantly illustrates how so many of us go wrong in relationships and in life through having the wrong mindsets – and how powerfully we can live when we have the right mindsets.

CHAPTER 22

BONUSES TO SUPERCHARGE YOUR CONFIDENCE & SUCCESS

As a thank you for coming on this journey with me and as a reward to you for going on your journey to becoming your best self, I have some bonuses I want to offer you.

Just go to the link below and you can get all the bonuses there:

www.unstoppableselfconfidence.com/bookbonuses

Here's what you'll get:

(Note: While I may change these from time to time, these are some of the best tools available for supercharging you on the journey to the life that you desire.)

- **30% discount on the audio version of the book** – I have personally found that the audio versions of my favorite self-help books to be incredibly powerful tools for accelerating my success. Listening to the wisdom they contain while I am walking along, driving, at the gym, or even just day to day is invaluable.

- **7 Day Confidence Masterclass** – To help you accelerate your journey to unstoppable, unshakable self-confidence, I have created a 7 Day Confidence Masterclass which has been used by thousands of people to transform their confidence fast. This is an on-demand video program, that you can go through at your own pace and contains structured lessons over 7 days to help you see big changes in your confidence fast.

- **Free 30 Minute Private Consultation Call** – If you'd like my and my team's help, we can offer you a free 30 minute private consultation call. We'll talk through your current situation and create a plan to help you see changes fast. Then we will show you what we can do for you, based on your specific situation, and then you can decide whether or not you want to become one of our success stories.

ABOUT THE AUTHOR

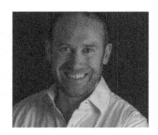

Andrew Leedham

After finding himself at his absolute lowest point, Andrew went on a mission to discover the secrets to creating the unstoppable self-confidence of the 1%.

What he discovered shocked him.

That most teaching on confidence and success was not only wrong but completely backwards and so ended up being destructive instead of beneficial.

And that with the secrets he discovered, he found that anyone could transform their confidence and success – permanently and FAST.

Through two brilliant mentors, Andrew learned the secrets of the mindset of the 1%. He learned that change isn't difficult and doesn't have to take a long time. He learned that confidence and success are a choice available to anyone.

Andrew's mission is to share these secrets with anyone who wants to learn and transform their sense of themselves and their success in life.

Andrew lives in the UK with his two wonderful, inspiring daughters, Lara and Ava.

Made in the USA
Las Vegas, NV
11 May 2023

71854190R00249